274-3843 Karen McIsaac

HANDBOOK OF EMERGENCY CARDIOVASCULAR CARE for Healthcare Providers

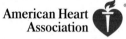

HEART & STROKE FOUNDATION OF CANADA
Finding answers. For life.

American Heart Association
Learn and Live

Editors

Mary Fran Hazinski, RN, MSN
John M. Field, MD
David Gilmore, MD

Reviewed by the members of

Committee on Emergency Cardiovascular Care
Subcommittee on Basic Life Support
Subcommittee on Pediatric Resuscitation
Subcommittee on Advanced Cardiovascular Life Support

With materials adapted from

International Guidelines 2005
Basic Life Support for Healthcare Providers
Pediatric Basic Life Support
Pediatric Advanced Life Support
Neonatal Resuscitation Textbook
Advanced Cardiovascular Life Support
ILCOR Advisory Statements
ACC/AHA Guidelines for Management
of ACS (2002-2007)

Additional contributions from

Anthony J. Busti, PharmD, BCPS
Louis Gonzales, NREMT-P
Alan Jay Schwartz, MD, MEd

© 2008 American Heart Association   ISBN 978-1-896242-30-9

Y0-BTE-806

i

Preface

This edition of the ECC Handbook provides our readers with the latest consensus recommendations from the 2005 International Consensus Conference on Cardiopulmonary Resuscitation and Emergency Cardiovascular Care Science, with new content developed since the publication of the 2005 Guidlines. The material in this handbook was selected for its relevance to patient care and its application to a quick-reference format.

For cardiac arrest, we strive to prevent when possible, treat effectively when challenged, and support humanely when death is imminent. In honor of your efforts we dedicate this book.

Mary Fran Hazinski
John M. Field
David A. Gilmore

Note on Medication Doses

Emergency cardiovascular care is a dynamic science. Advances in treatment and drug therapies occur rapidly. Readers are advised to check for changes in recommended dose, indications, and contraindications in the following sources: *Currents in Emergency Cardiovascular Care*, future editions of this handbook, and the AHA textbooks as well as the package insert product information sheet for each drug.

Clinical condition and pharmacokinetics may require drug dose or interval dosing adjustments. Specific parameters may require monitoring, for example, creatinine clearance or QT interval.

Some medications listed in this handbook were scientifically reviewed by the Guidelines evidence-based evaluation process. They may not be available in all countries and may not be specifically approved by the FDA for a particular treatment or application.

Copyright Notice

Evidence-Based Resuscitation Guidelines

In 1999, 2000, and in 2005, more than 300 international resuscitation experts met to evaluate published articles and develop evidence-based recommendations for CPR and emergency cardiovascular care. The definitions used for the Classes of Recommendation in 2005 are listed below.

Levels of Evidence

Evidence	Definition
Level 1	Randomized clinical trials or meta-analyses of multiple clinical trials with substantial treatment effects
Level 2	Randomized clinical trials with smaller or less significant treatment effects
Level 3	Prospective, controlled, non-randomized, cohort studies
Level 4	Historic, non-randomized, cohort or case-control studies
Level 5	Case series; patients compiled in serial fashion, lacking a control group
Level 6	Animal studies or mechanical model studies
Level 7	Extrapolations from existing data collected for other purposes, theoretical analyses
Level 8	Rational conjecture (common sense); common practices accepted before evidence-based guidelines

Applying Classification of Recommendations and Level of Evidence

Class I	**Benefit >>>Risk**	Procedure/treatment or diagnostic test/assessment should be performed/administered.
Class IIa	**Benefit >>Risk**	It is reasonable to perform procedure/administer treatment or perform diagnostic test/assessment.
Class IIb	**Benefit ≥Risk**	Procedure/treatment or diagnostic test/assessment may be considered.
Class III	**Risk ≥Benefit**	Procedure/treatment or diagnostic test/assessment should NOT be performed/administered. It is not helpful and may be harmful.
Class Indeterminate		• Research just getting started. • Continuing area of research. • No recommendations until further research (eg, cannot recommend for or against).

Contents

Basic Life Support

Advanced Cardiovascular Life Support

Newborn Resuscitation

Pediatric Advanced Life Support

CPR/Rescue Breathing

Establish unresponsiveness
Activate EMS system or appropriate resuscitation team at appropriate time.

A. Open airway
Head tilt–chin lift or jaw thrust.

B. Check for breathing
Look, listen, feel for no more than 10 seconds.
- *If victim is breathing* or resumes effective breathing, place in the recovery position.
- *If victim is not breathing,* give 2 breaths that make chest rise using pocket mask or bag mask. Release completely, allow for exhalation between breaths.

C. HCP: Pulse check.
Check for pulse for no more than 10 seconds (carotid in child and adult; brachial or femoral in infant).

Summary of BLS ABCD Maneuvers for Infants, Children, and Adults (Newborn information not included)

Note: Maneuvers used by only Healthcare Providers are indicated by "HCP."

Maneuver	Adult	Child	Infant
	Lay rescuer: ≥8 years HCP: Adolescent and older	Lay rescuers: 1-8 years HCP: 1 year to adolescent	Under 1 year of age
Airway	Head tilt–chin lift (HCP: Suspected trauma, use jaw thrust)		
Breaths Initial	2 breaths at 1 second per breath	2 effective breaths (make chest rise) at 1 second per breath	
HCP: Rescue breathing without chest compressions	10 to 12/minute (approximately 1 breath every 5 to 6 seconds)	12 to 20/minute (approximately 1 breath every 3 to 5 seconds)	
HCP: Rescue breaths for CPR with advanced airway	8 to 10/minute (approximately 1 breath every 6 to 8 seconds)		
Foreign-body airway obstruction for responsive victim	Abdominal thrusts		Back slaps and chest thrusts

- *If pulse present but breathing is absent,* provide rescue breathing 1 breath every 5 to 6 seconds for adult, 1 breath every 3 to 5 seconds for infant or child. Recheck pulse about every 2 minutes.
- *If pulse absent:* Begin chest compressions if no definite pulse after 10 seconds; cycles of 30 compressions and 2 breaths until AED or ALS providers arrive.
- *If pulse present but <60 per minute in infant or child with poor perfusion:* Begin chest compressions.

Continue basic life support
Integrate newborn resuscitation, pediatric advanced life support, or advanced cardiovascular life support at earliest opportunity.

D. Defibrillation
Defibrillation using automated external defibrillators (AEDs) is an integral part of basic life support.

Circulation HCP: Pulse check (≤10 sec)	Carotid (HCP can use femoral in child)		Brachial or femoral
Compression landmarks	Center of chest, between nipples (Child: Lower half of sternum)		Just below nipple line
Compression method: Push hard and fast, allow complete recoil	Heel of one hand, other hand on top	2 hands: Heel of 1 hand, with second on top or 1 hand: Heel of 1 hand only	2 fingers HCP (2 rescuers): 2 thumb–encircling hands
Compression depth	1½ to 2 inches	Approximately one third to one half the depth of the chest	
Compression rate	Approximately 100/minute		
Compression-ventilation ratio	30:2 (1 and 2 rescuers)	30:2 (single rescuer) HCP: 15:2 (2 rescuers)	
Defibrillation AED	Use adult pads. Do not use child pads.	Use AED after about 2 minutes of CPR (out of hospital). Use pediatric system for child 1 to 8 years if available; if not, use adult system. HCP: For sudden collapse (out of hospital) or in-hospital arrest, use AED as soon as possible.	No recommendation for infants <1 year of age

Relief of Foreign-Body Airway Obstruction and Recovery Position

Adult
(Adolescent [puberty] and older)
1. Ask "Are you choking?"
2. Give abdominal thrusts/Heimlich maneuver or chest thrusts for pregnant or obese victims.
3. Repeat abdominal thrusts until effective or victim becomes unresponsive.

Victim becomes unresponsive
4. Activate EMS. If second rescuer is present, send that person to activate EMS system.
5. Begin CPR.
6. Look into mouth when opening the airway during CPR. Use finger sweep only to remove visible foreign body in unresponsive victim.
7. Continue CPR until ALS arrives.

Child
(1 year to adolescent [puberty])
1. Ask "Are you choking?"
2. Give abdominal thrusts/Heimlich maneuver.
3. Repeat abdominal thrusts until effective or victim becomes unresponsive.

Victim becomes unresponsive
4. If second rescuer is present, send that person to activate EMS system.
5. Begin CPR.
6. Look into mouth when opening the airway during CPR. Use finger sweep only to remove visible foreign body in unresponsive victim.
7. Continue CPR for 5 cycles or 2 minutes and then activate EMS system. Return to child and continue CPR until ALS arrives.

Infant
(Less than 1 year of age)
1. Confirm severe airway obstruction. Check for the sudden onset of severe breathing difficulty, ineffective or silent cough, weak or silent cry.
2. Give up to 5 back slaps *and* up to 5 chest thrusts.
3. Repeat step 2 until effective or victim becomes unresponsive.

Victim becomes unresponsive
4. If second rescuer is present, send that person to activate EMS system.
5. Begin CPR.
6. Look into mouth when opening the airway during CPR. Use finger sweep only to remove visible foreign body in unresponsive victim.
7. Continue CPR for 5 cycles or 2 minutes and then activate EMS system. Return to infant and continue CPR until ALS arrives.

During ventilation attempts use appropriate size mask or bag mask as soon as available. Activate resuscitation team as soon as possible. Supplementary oxygen delivery equipment should be immediately available. Consider forceps, cricotomy/transtracheal catheter ventilation. Refer to *BLS for Healthcare Providers* for more complete discussions of topics related to foreign-body airway obstruction.

Recovery Position

If the victim is not injured but is unresponsive with adequate breathing and a pulse, turn the victim on his or her side in the recovery position. This position keeps the airway open. No single recovery position is perfect for all victims. The position should be a stable lateral position so that the tongue does not block the airway and fluid can drain from the mouth. The victim's spine should be straight. Position the arms to avoid compression of the chest and the dependent arm.

The illustrations below show one technique for placement of a patient in an acceptable recovery position. If the victim stops breathing, turn the victim supine and provide rescue breathing or other steps of CPR as needed.

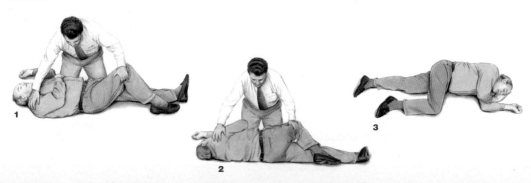

Recommendations for CPR Before Insertion of an Advanced Airway

During 2-rescuer CPR when there is no advanced airway in place, rescuers perform cycles of 30 compressions and 2 breaths. The compressor pauses after every 30 compressions to allow delivery of 2 rescue breaths. Rescuers should change compressor role every 5 cycles or 2 minutes. Rescuers should attempt to accomplish any change in compressor role in less than 5 seconds.

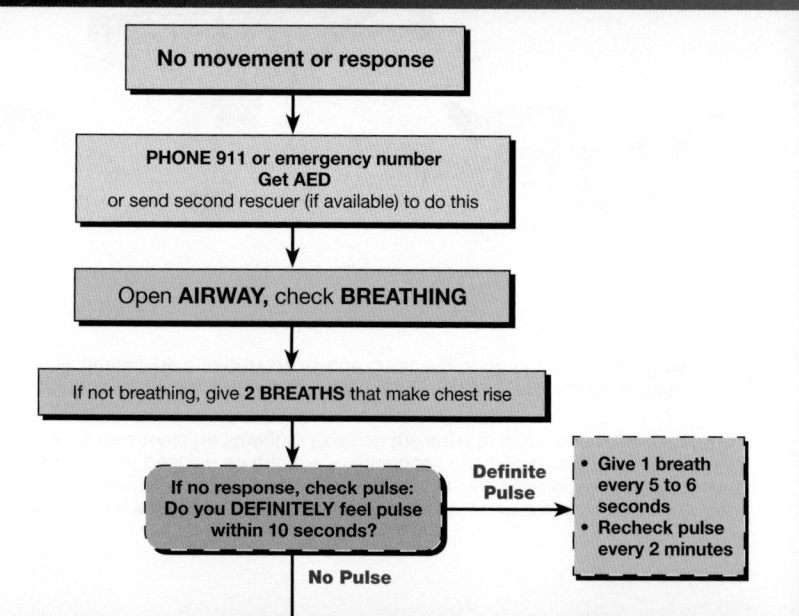

Recommendations for CPR After Insertion of an Advanced Airway*

Once an advanced airway is in place, 2 rescuers no longer deliver "cycles" of CPR (compressions interrupted by pauses for ventilation). Instead, the compressing rescuer should give continuous chest compressions at a rate of 100 per minute without pauses for ventilation. The rescuer delivering ventilation provides 1 breath every 6 to 8 seconds. Two or more rescuers should change compressor role approximately every 2 minutes to prevent compressor fatigue and deterioration in quality and rate of chest compressions. Rescuers should attempt to accomplish any change in compressor role in less than 5 seconds.

Give cycles of 30 COMPRESSIONS and 2 BREATHS until AED/defibrillator arrives, ALS providers take over, or victim starts to move
Push hard and fast (100/min) and release completely
Minimize interruptions in compressions

↓

AED/defibrillator ARRIVES

↓

Check rhythm
Shockable rhythm?

Shockable

Give 1 shock
Resume CPR immediately
for 5 cycles

Not Shockable

Resume CPR immediately
for 5 cycles
Check rhythm every 5 cycles; continue until ALS providers take over or victim starts to move

*Advanced Airway = endotrachial tube, laryngeal mask airway (LMA), Combitube

Lay Rescuer AED Programs

Lay rescuer automated external defibrillation (AED) programs improve survival from out-of-hospital cardiac arrest by placing AEDs throughout the community and training lay rescuers in CPR and use of the AED. The Heart and Stroke Foundation has resources developed for lay rescuer AED program directors. For more information, contact your provincial HSF office at 1-888-HSF-INFO (1-888-473-4636) or go to **www.heartandstroke.ca.**

Background

- Immediate bystander CPR and defibrillation within 3 to 5 minutes of collapse have resulted in survival rates of 41% to 74% for victims of witnessed VF arrest in airports, casinos, and first-responder programs with police officers.

  — Immediate bystander CPR can double the VF survival rate at any interval to defibrillation.
  — Early CPR and early defibrillation with AEDs can double survival over that resulting from early CPR alone.

- Lay rescuer AED programs must be carefully planned, with a practiced response and a process of continuous quality improvement. The program must reduce the interval from collapse to initiation of bystander CPR and from collapse to defibrillation.

- Lay rescuers who use AEDs in a CPR effort are protected by provincial Good Samaritan/emergency medical act legislation. Contact your provincial ministry of health for more information about Good Samaritan/emergency medical act legislation in your province.

Preprogram Planning

- The program coordinator should establish a link with the EMS system personnel and invite their involvement.

- The program coordinator should determine the number and location of AEDs. AEDs should be placed near a telephone (to facilitate EMS notification) and be no more than a brisk 1-minute to 1½ -minute walk from any location. Programs will have the greatest potential to save lives if they are created in locations where sudden cardiac arrest is likely to occur (eg, sites with >250 adults over 50 years of age present for >16 h/day).

Critical Program Elements

1. **Program oversight by a healthcare provider**
   - A planned and practiced response; typically this requires oversight by a healthcare provider.

2. **Training of anticipated rescuers in CPR and use of the AED**
   - Anticipated rescuers should be prepared to recognize emergencies, phone 911, retrieve AED, begin CPR immediately, and use AED.

3. **Link with the local EMS system**
   - Notify EMS system personnel about establishment of AED program.
   - Notify EMS dispatcher of location and type of AED on premises.

4. **Process of continuous quality improvement**
   - It is reasonable for lay rescuer AED programs to implement a process of continuous quality improvement programs. Quality improvement efforts for lay rescuer AED programs should use both routine inspections and postevent data from AED recordings and responder reports.
   - Performance of an emergency response plan, including accurate time intervals for key interventions (collapse to shock or no shock advisory to initiation of CPR) and patient outcome.
   - Responder performance.
   - AED function, including accuracy of the ECG rhythm analysis.
   - Battery status and function.
   - Electrode pad function and readiness, including expiration date.

The Primary-Secondary Survey Approach to Emergency Cardiovascular Care

The **ACLS Provider Course** teaches the **Primary and Secondary Surveys** approach for emergency cardiovascular care. This memory aid describes the 2 surveys using forms of the "ABCD" memory aid. At each step the responder performs an assessment, manages problems detected, and evaluates the response to therapy.

The BLS Primary Survey

Assess	Management
Airway *–Is the airway open?*	Open the airway using noninvasive techniques (head tilt–chin lift or jaw thrust without head extension if trauma is suspected).
Breathing *–Is the patient breathing and are respirations adequate?*	Look, listen, and feel for adequate breathing. Give 2 rescue breaths. Give each breath over 1 second. Each breath should make the chest rise. Do not ventilate too fast (rate) or too much (volume).
Circulation *–Is a pulse present?*	Check carotid pulse for at least 5 seconds but no longer than 10 seconds. Perform high-quality CPR until an AED arrives.
Defibrillation *–If no pulse, check for a shock-able rhythm with a manual defibrillator or use an AED.*	• Provide shocks as indicated. • Follow each shock immediately with CPR, beginning with chest compressions.

(continued)

The ACLS Secondary Survey

Assess	Action as Appropriate
Airway –Is the airway patent? –Is an advanced airway indicated?	• Maintain airway patency in unconscious patients by use of head tilt–chin lift, oropharyngeal airway (OPA), or nasopharyngeal airway (NPA). • Use advanced airway management if needed (eg, LMA, Combitube, endotracheal intubation).

Breathing
–Are oxygenation and ventilation adequate?
 	
–Is an advanced airway indicated?
 	
–Is proper placement of airway device confirmed?
 	
–Is tube secured and placement reconfirmed frequently?
 	
–Are exhaled CO_2 and oxyhemoglobin saturation monitored?
	• Give supplementary oxygen.
	• Assess the adequacy of oxygenation and ventilation by
	  — Clinical criteria (chest rise)
	  — Oxygen saturation
	  — Capnometry or capnography
	
	The benefit of advanced airway placement is weighed against the adverse effect of interrupting chest compressions. If bag-mask ventilation is adequate, insertion of an advanced airway may be deferred until the patient fails to respond to initial CPR and defibrillation or until spontaneous circulation returns.
	If advanced airway devices are used:
	
	• Confirm proper integration of CPR and ventilation.
	• Confirm proper placement of advanced airway devices by
	  — Physical examination
	  — Measurement of exhaled CO_2
	  — Use of esophageal detector device
	• Secure the device to prevent dislodgment.
	• Continue exhaled CO_2 measurement.

The ACLS Secondary Survey	
Circulation –What was the initial cardiac rhythm? –What is the current cardiac rhythm? –Have you established access for drug and fluid administration? –Does the patient need volume (fluid) for resuscitation? –Are medications needed for rhythm or blood pressure?	• Obtain IV/IO access. • Attach ECG leads and monitor for arrhythmias or cardiac arrest rhythms (eg, VF, pulseless VT, asystole, and PEA). • Give appropriate drugs to manage rhythm (eg, amiodarone, lidocaine, atropine, magnesium) and blood pressure (eg, epinephrine, vasopressin, and dopamine). • Give IV/IO fluids if needed.
Differential **D**iagnosis –Why did this patient develop cardiac arrest? –Why is the patient still in arrest? –Can we identify a reversible cause of this arrest?	• Search for, find, and treat reversible causes (ie, definitive care).

Pulseless Arrest Algorithm

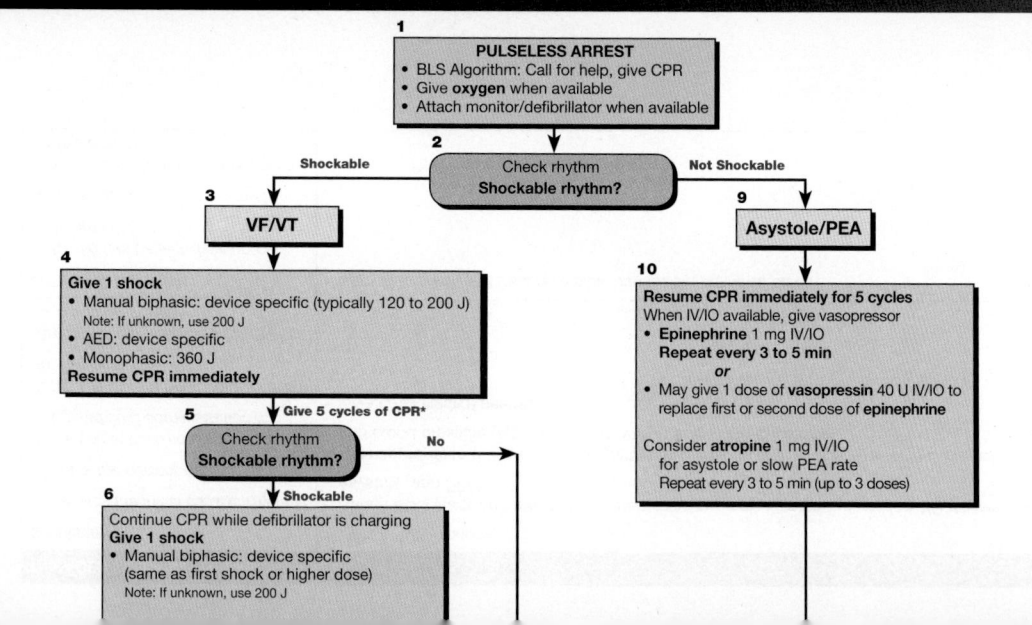

1

PULSELESS ARREST
- BLS Algorithm: Call for help, give CPR
- Give **oxygen** when available
- Attach monitor/defibrillator when available

2

Shockable ←——— Check rhythm **Shockable rhythm?** ———→ Not Shockable

3

VF/VT

9

Asystole/PEA

4

Give 1 shock
- Manual biphasic: device specific (typically 120 to 200 J)
  Note: If unknown, use 200 J
- AED: device specific
- Monophasic: 360 J
Resume CPR immediately

10

Resume CPR immediately for 5 cycles
When IV/IO available, give vasopressor
- **Epinephrine** 1 mg IV/IO
  Repeat every 3 to 5 min
  or
- May give 1 dose of **vasopressin** 40 U IV/IO to replace first or second dose of **epinephrine**

Consider **atropine** 1 mg IV/IO
for asystole or slow PEA rate
Repeat every 3 to 5 min (up to 3 doses)

Give 5 cycles of CPR*

5

Check rhythm **Shockable rhythm?** ———→ No

Shockable

6

Continue CPR while defibrillator is charging
Give 1 shock
- Manual biphasic: device specific (same as first shock or higher dose)
  Note: If unknown, use 200 J

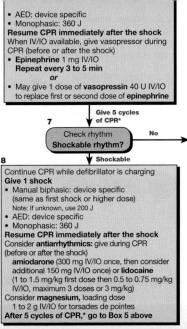

- AED: device specific
- Monophasic: 360 J

Resume CPR immediately after the shock
When IV/IO available, give vasopressor during CPR (before or after the shock)
- **Epinephrine** 1 mg IV/IO
  Repeat every 3 to 5 min
  or
- May give 1 dose of **vasopressin** 40 U IV/IO to replace first or second dose of **epinephrine**

7

Give 5 cycles of CPR*

Check rhythm
Shockable rhythm?

No →

8

Continue CPR while defibrillator is charging
Give 1 shock
- Manual biphasic: device specific (same as first shock or higher dose)
  Note: If unknown, use 200 J
- AED: device specific
- Monophasic: 360 J

Resume CPR immediately after the shock
Consider antiarrhythmics: give during CPR (before or after the shock)
  amiodarone (300 mg IV/IO once, then consider additional 150 mg IV/IO once) or **lidocaine** (1 to 1.5 mg/kg first dose then 0.5 to 0.75 mg/kg IV/IO, maximum 3 doses or 3 mg/kg)
Consider **magnesium**, loading dose 1 to 2 g IV/IO for torsades de pointes
After 5 cycles of CPR,* go to Box 5 above

Shockable ↓

12

- If asystole, go to Box 10
- If electrical activity, check pulse. If no pulse, go to Box 10
- If pulse present, begin postresuscitation care

11

Give 5 cycles of CPR*

Check rhythm
Shockable rhythm?

Not Shockable ← → Shockable

13

Go to Box 4

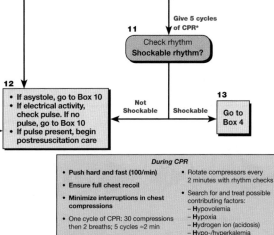

During CPR

- **Push hard and fast (100/min)**
- **Ensure full chest recoil**
- **Minimize interruptions in chest compressions**
- One cycle of CPR: 30 compressions then 2 breaths; 5 cycles ≈2 min
- Avoid hyperventilation
- Secure airway and confirm placement
- *After an advanced airway is placed, rescuers no longer deliver "cycles" of CPR. Give continuous chest compressions without pauses for breaths. Give 8 to 10 breaths/minute. Check rhythm every 2 minutes.

- Rotate compressors every 2 minutes with rhythm checks
- Search for and treat possible contributing factors:
  – Hypovolemia
  – Hypoxia
  – Hydrogen ion (acidosis)
  – Hypo-/hyperkalemia
  – Hypoglycemia
  – Hypothermia
  – Toxins
  – Tamponade, cardiac
  – Tension pneumothorax
  – Thrombosis (coronary or pulmonary)
  – Trauma

A. Ventricular Fibrillation/Pulseless VT

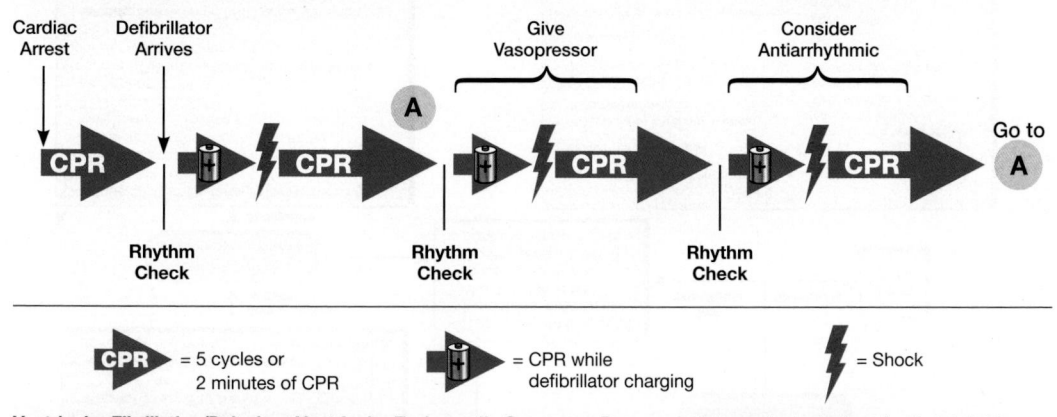

Ventricular Fibrillation/Pulseless Ventricular Tachycardia Sequence: Prepare next drug prior to rhythm check. Administer drug during CPR, as soon as possible after the rhythm check confirms VF/pulseless VT. Do not delay shock. Continue CPR while drugs are prepared and administered and defibrillator is charging. Ideally, chest compressions should be interrupted only for ventilation (until advanced airway placed), rhythm check, and actual shock delivery.

B. Asystole and Pulseless Electrical Activity

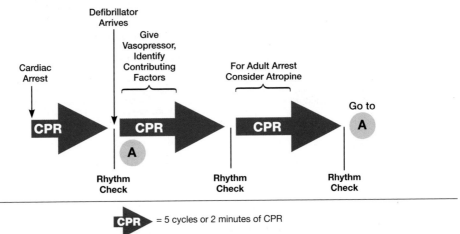

CPR ▶ = 5 cycles or 2 minutes of CPR

ACLS and PALS Treatment of Asystole and Pulseless Electrical Activity (PEA) Sequence: Prepare next drug prior to rhythm check. Administer drug during CPR, as soon as possible after the rhythm check confirms no VF/pulseless VT. Continue CPR while drugs are prepared and administered. Ideally, chest compressions should be interrupted only for ventilation (until advanced airway placed) and rhythm check. Search for and treat possible contributing factors.

Using Conventional (Manual) Defibrillators (Monophasic or Biphasic)

1. Turn on defibrillator. Select energy level at 360 J for monophasic manual defibrillator. Select device-specific energy level for biphasic manual defibrillator, typically 120 to 200 J; if unknown select 200 J.
2. Set "lead select" switch on "paddles" (or lead I, II, or III if monitor leads are used).
3. Apply adhesive electrodes or if using paddles, apply gel to paddles or position conductor pads on patient's chest.
4. Position paddles or remote defibrillation pads on patient (sternum-apex).
5. Visually check the monitor display and assess the rhythm. (Subsequent steps assume VF/VT is present—perform steps to minimize interruptions in chest compressions.)
6. Announce to the team members, "Charging defibrillator!"
7. Press "charge" button on apex paddle or defibrillator controls.
8. When the defibrillator is fully charged, state firmly in a forceful voice the following chant (or suitable equivalent) before each shock (this chant should take about 5 seconds total):
   - *"I am going to shock on three. One, I'm clear."* (Check to make sure you are clear of contact with the patient, the stretcher, and the equipment.)
   - *"Two, you're clear."* (Make a visual check to ensure that no one continues to touch the patient or stretcher. In particular, check the person providing ventilations. That person's hands should not be touching the ventilatory adjuncts, including the endotracheal tube! Be sure oxygen is not flowing across the patient's chest. Turn oxygen off or direct flow away from the patient's chest.)
   - *"Three, everybody's clear."* (Check yourself one more time before pressing the "shock" buttons.)
9. Pads are preferred; if paddles are used, apply 25 pounds of pressure.
10. Press the "shock" button on the defibrillator or press the two paddle "discharge" buttons simultaneously after confirming all personnel are clear of the patient.
11. Immediately resume CPR, beginning with compressions, for 5 cycles (about 2 minutes), then recheck rhythm. Interruption of CPR should be brief.
12. Shock at 360 J for monophasic manual defibrillator. Select device-specific energy for biphasic manual defibrillator, typically 120 to 200 J; if unknown use 200 J.

Using Automated External Defibrillators (AEDs)

Provide CPR until AED arrives. Minimize interruptions in CPR (eg, to analyze rhythm, deliver shock). Keep interruptions as short as possible. All AEDs operate using the following basic steps.

1. POWER ON	• Open the carrying case or the top of the AED. • Turn the power on (some devices will "power on" automatically when you open the lid or case).

2. Attach electrode pads to the patient's bare chest	Choose correct pads (adult vs child) for size/age of the patient. Use child pads or a child system for children less than 8 years of age if available. ***Do not use child pads or a child system for patients 8 years and older.***
	• Peel the backing away from the electrode pads.
	• Quickly wipe the patient's chest if it is covered with water or sweat.
	• Attach the adhesive electrode pads to the patient's bare chest.
	   — Place one electrode pad on the upper-right side of the bare chest to the right of the breastbone directly below the collarbone.
	   — Place the other pad to the left of the nipple, with the top margin of the pad a few inches below the left armpit.
	• Attach the AED connecting cables to the AED box (some are preconnected).

3. Analyze the rhythm.	• Always clear the patient during analysis. Be sure no one is touching the victim, not even the person in charge of giving breaths. • Some AEDs will instruct you to push a button to allow the AED to begin analyzing the heart rhythm; others will do that automatically. The AED rhythm analysis may take about 5 to 15 seconds. • The AED then instructs whether or not a shock is needed.
4. If the AED advises a **shock,** it will tell you to **be sure to clear the patient.**	• Clear the patient before delivering the shock; be sure no one is touching the patient. • Loudly state a "clear the patient" message, such as "I'm clear, you're clear, everybody's clear" or simply "Clear." • Perform a visual check to ensure that no one is in contact with the patient. • Press the SHOCK button. • The shock will produce a sudden contraction of the patient's muscles.

As soon as the shock is delivered, resume CPR, starting with chest compressions, with cycles of compressions and breaths at a 30:2 ratio. Do not perform a pulse or rhythm check. After 2 minutes of CPR, the AED will prompt you to repeat steps 3 and 4.

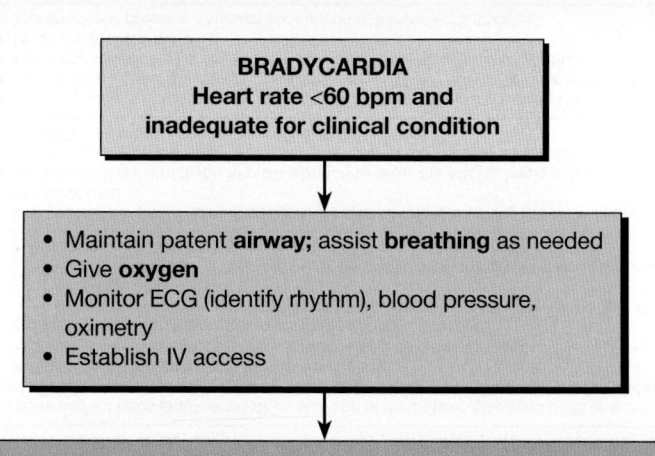

BRADYCARDIA
Heart rate <60 bpm and
inadequate for clinical condition

- Maintain patent **airway;** assist **breathing** as needed
- Give **oxygen**
- Monitor ECG (identify rhythm), blood pressure, oximetry
- Establish IV access

Signs or symptoms of poor perfusion caused by the bradycardia?
(eg, acute altered mental status, ongoing chest pain, hypotension or other signs of shock)

Observe/Monitor ← **Adequate Perfusion** | **Poor Perfusion** →

- **Prepare for transcutaneous pacing;** use without delay for high-degree block (type II second-degree block or third-degree AV block)
- Consider **atropine** 0.5 mg IV while awaiting pacer. May repeat to a total dose of 3 mg. If ineffective, begin pacing
- Consider **epinephrine** (2 to 10 μg/min) or **dopamine** (2 to 10 μg/kg per minute) infusion while awaiting pacer or if pacing ineffective

↓

- Prepare for **transvenous pacing**
- Treat contributing causes
- Consider expert consultation

Reminders

- If pulseless arrest develops, go to Pulseless Arrest Algorithm
- Search for and treat possible contributing factors:
  - **H**ypovolemia
  - **H**ypoxia
  - **H**ydrogen ion (acidosis)
  - **H**ypo-/hyperkalemia
  - **H**ypoglycemia
  - **H**ypothermia
  - **T**oxins
  - **T**amponade, cardiac
  - **T**ension pneumothorax
  - **T**hrombosis (coronary or pulmonary)
  - **T**rauma (hypovolemia, increased ICP)

10

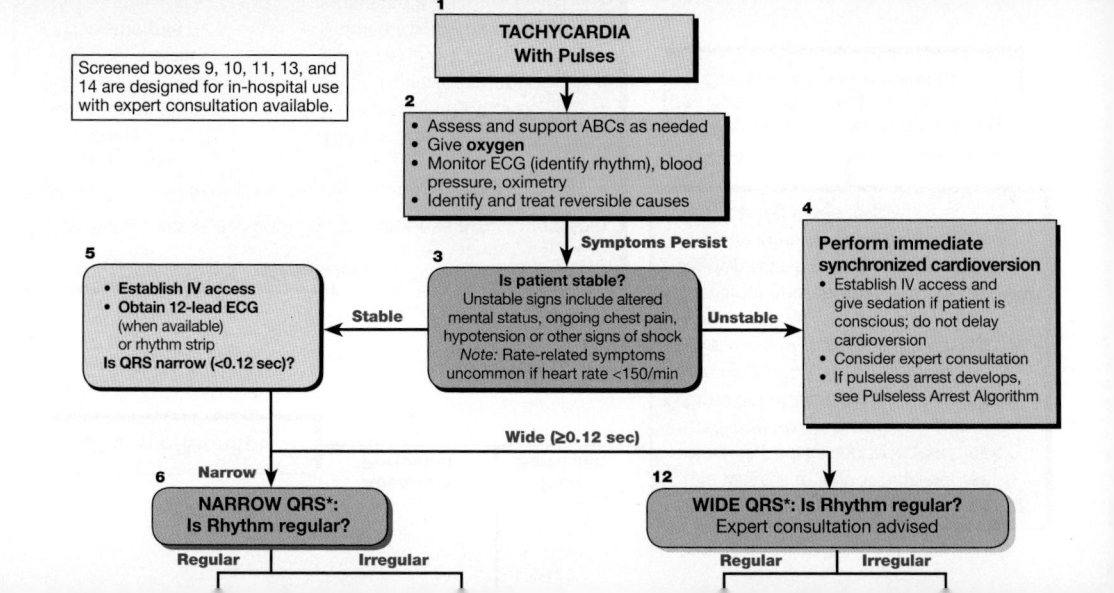

Screened boxes 9, 10, 11, 13, and 14 are designed for in-hospital use with expert consultation available.

1
TACHYCARDIA
With Pulses

2
- Assess and support ABCs as needed
- Give **oxygen**
- Monitor ECG (identify rhythm), blood pressure, oximetry
- Identify and treat reversible causes

Symptoms Persist

4
Perform immediate synchronized cardioversion
- Establish IV access and give sedation if patient is conscious; do not delay cardioversion
- Consider expert consultation
- If pulseless arrest develops, see Pulseless Arrest Algorithm

5
- Establish IV access
- Obtain 12-lead ECG (when available) or rhythm strip
Is QRS narrow (<0.12 sec)?

Stable

3
Is patient stable?
Unstable signs include altered mental status, ongoing chest pain, hypotension or other signs of shock
Note: Rate-related symptoms uncommon if heart rate <150/min

Unstable

Wide (≥0.12 sec)

6
Narrow
NARROW QRS*:
Is Rhythm regular?

Regular   Irregular

12
WIDE QRS*: Is Rhythm regular?
Expert consultation advised

Regular   Irregular

7

- Attempt vagal maneuvers
- Give **adenosine** 6 mg rapid IV push. If no conversion, give 12 mg rapid IV push; may repeat 12 mg dose once

8

Does rhythm convert?
Note: Consider expert consultation

Converts | **Does Not Convert**

9

If rhythm converts, probable reentry SVT (reentry supraventricular tachycardia):

- Observe for recurrence
- Treat recurrence with **adenosine** or longer-acting AV nodal blocking agents (eg, **diltiazem**, **β-blockers**)

10

If rhythm does NOT convert, possible **atrial flutter**, **ectopic atrial tachycardia**, or **junctional tachycardia**:

- Control rate (eg, **diltiazem**, **β-blockers**; use β-blockers with caution in pulmonary disease or CHF)
- Treat underlying cause
- Consider expert consultation

*Note: If patient becomes unstable, go to Box 4.

11

Irregular Narrow-Complex Tachycardia
Probable **atrial fibrillation** or possible **atrial flutter** or **MAT** (multifocal atrial tachycardia)

- Consider expert consultation
- Control rate (eg, **diltiazem**, **β-blockers**; use β-blockers with caution in pulmonary disease or CHF)

13

If ventricular tachycardia or uncertain rhythm

- **Amiodarone**
  150 mg IV over 10 min
  Repeat as needed to maximum dose of 2.2 g/24 hours
- Prepare for elective **synchronized cardioversion**

If SVT with aberrancy

- Give **adenosine** (go to Box 7)

14

If atrial fibrillation with aberrancy

- See Irregular Narrow-Complex Tachycardia (Box 11)

If pre-excited atrial fibrillation (AF + WPW)

- Expert consultation advised
- Avoid AV nodal blocking agents (eg, **adenosine**, **digoxin**, **diltiazem**, **verapamil**)
- Consider antiarrhythmics (eg, **amiodarone** 150 mg IV over 10 min)

If recurrent polymorphic VT, seek expert consultation

If torsades de pointes, give **magnesium** (load with 1-2 g over 5-60 min, then infusion)

During Evaluation

- Secure, verify airway and vascular access when possible
- Consider expert consultation
- Prepare for cardioversion

Treat possible contributing factors:

- **H**ypovolemia
- **H**ypoxia
- **H**ydrogen ion (acidosis)
- **H**ypo-/hyperkalemia
- **H**ypoglycemia
- **H**ypothermia

- **T**oxins
- **T**amponade, cardiac
- **T**ension pneumothorax
- **T**hrombosis (coronary or pulmonary)
- **T**rauma (hypovolemia)

Rhythm strips A and B demonstrate the requirement to evaluate the QT interval in light of the heart rate. Strip C depicts an ECG from a patient with a prolonged QT interval:

- *Strip A:* A bradycardic rhythm of 57 bpm has a QT interval of 0.4 second, which is less than the upper limit of normal for a rate of 57 (0.41 second for a man), and a QT/RR ratio of 38% (<40%).

- *Strip B:* A faster rate of 78 bpm has a shorter measured QT interval of 0.24 second (faster-shorter/slower-longer), which is less than the upper limit of normal for a rate of 78 (0.35 second for a man), and a QT/RR ratio of 33% (<40%).

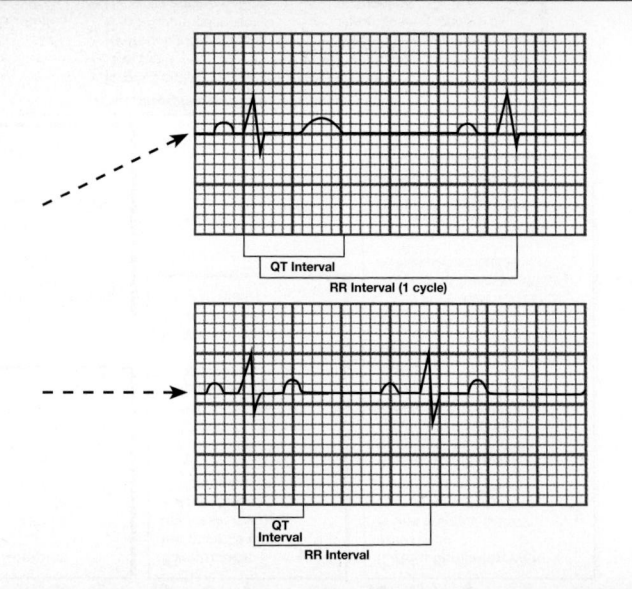

- *Strip C:* Here the QT interval is prolonged at 0.45 second, exceeding the upper limit of normal for a rate of 80 bpm (0.34 second for a man and 0.37 second for a woman). The QT/RR ratio of 59% is considerably above the 40% rule of thumb. This strip is from a patient who took an overdose of a tricyclic antidepressant.

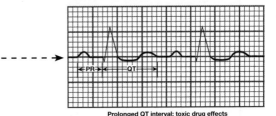

Prolonged QT interval: toxic drug effects

Parameter	Rhythm Strip A	Rhythm Strip B	Rhythm Strip C
Rate	57 bpm	78 bpm	80 bpm
RR interval (cardiac cycle time)	1.04 seconds (26 x 1-mm boxes)	0.72 second (18 x 1-mm boxes)	0.76 second (19 x 1-mm boxes)
QT interval, measured	0.4 second (10 x 1-mm boxes)	0.24 second (6 x 1-mm boxes)	0.45 second (11 x 1-mm boxes)
QT$_c$ interval: QT interval corrected for heart rate (upper limit of normal QT interval range for a man or a woman from Table on next page)	0.41 second (man) 0.45 second (woman)	0.35 second (man) 0.38 second (woman)	0.34 second (man) 0.37 second (woman)
QT/RR ratio: QT interval divided by RR interval	38% (0.4/1.04 = 0.384)	33% (0.24/0.72 = 0.333)	59% (0.45/0.76 = 0.592)

Reprinted with permission from *ACLS Scenarios: Core Concepts for Case-Based Learning* by R.O. Cummins. Copyright 1996 Mosby, Inc.

Maximum QT Interval (Upper Limits of Normal) for Men and Women Based on Heart Rate

Note the relationship between decreasing heart rate and increasing maximum QT interval. For normal heart range of 60 to 100 per minute (grey), the maximum QT intervals for men and women (light blue) are less than one half the RR interval (marigold). Most people estimate QT and RR intervals by counting the number of 1-mm boxes and then multiplying by 0.04 second. The third column was added to eliminate the need to multiply by 0.04.

Heart Rate (per minute)	RR Interval (sec)	Upper Limits of Normal QT Interval (sec)	
(note decreasing)	Or "Cycle Time" (note increasing)	Men (note increasing)	Women (note increasing)
150	0.4	0.25	0.28
136	0.44	0.26	0.29
125	0.48	0.28	0.3
115	0.52	0.29	0.32
107	0.56	0.3	0.33
100	0.6	0.31	0.34
93	0.64	0.32	0.35
88	0.68	0.33	0.36

78	0.72	0.35	0.38
75	0.8	0.36	0.39
71	0.84	0.37	0.4
68	0.88	0.38	0.41
65	0.92	0.38	0.42
62	0.96	0.39	0.43
60	1	0.4	0.44
57	1.04	0.41	0.45
52	1.08	0.42	0.47
50	1.2	0.44	0.48

Tachycardia
With serious signs and symptoms related to the tachycardia

If ventricular rate is >150 bpm, prepare for **immediate cardioversion.** May give brief trial of medications based on specific arrhythmias. Immediate cardioversion is generally not needed if heart rate is ≤150 bpm.

Have available at bedside
- Oxygen saturation monitor
- Suction device
- IV line
- Intubation equipment

Steps for Synchronized Cardioversion

1. Consider sedation.
2. Turn on defibrillator (monophasic or biphasic).
3. Attach monitor leads to the patient ("white to right, red to ribs, what's left over to the left shoulder") and ensure proper display of the patient's rhythm.
4. Engage the synchronization mode by pressing the "sync" control button.
5. Look for markers on R waves indicating sync mode.
6. If necessary, adjust monitor gain until sync markers occur with each R wave.
7. Select appropriate energy level.
8. Position conductor pads on patient (or apply gel to paddles).
9. Position paddle on patient (sternum-apex).
10. Announce to team members:
    "Charging cardiovertor—stand clear!"
11. Press "charge" button on apex paddle (right hand).
12. When the cardioverter/defibrillator is charged, begin the final clearing chant. State firmly in a forceful voice the following chant before each shock:

```
          ▼
┌──────────────────────────────────────┐
│ Premedicate whenever possible¹       │
└──────────────────────────────────────┘
          ▼
```

Synchronized cardioversion[2-5]

If	Sequence
Atrial fibrillation	100 to 200 J, 300 J, 360 J
Stable monomorphic VT	100 J, 200 J, 300 J, 360 J
Other SVT, atrial flutter	50 J, 100 J, 200 J, 300 J, 360 J
Polymorphic VT (irregular form and rate) and unstable	Treat as VF with high-energy shock (defibrillation doses)

Notes:

1. Effective regimens have included a sedative (eg, *diazepam, midazolam, barbiturates, etomidate, ketamine, methohexital, propofol*) with or without an analgesic agent (eg, *fentanyl, morphine*). Many experts recommend anesthesia if service is readily available.
2. Biphasic waveforms using lower energy are acceptable if documented to be clinically equivalent or superior to reports of monophasic shock success. Extrapolation from elective cardioversion of atrial fibrillation supports an initial biphasic dose of 100 J to 120 J with escalation as needed. Consult the device manufacturer for specific recommendations.
3. Both monophasic and biphasic waveforms are acceptable if documented as clinically equivalent to reports of monophasic shock success.
4. Note possible need to resynchronize after each cardioversion.
5. If delays in synchronization occur and clinical condition is critical, go immediately to unsynchronized shocks.

- *"I am going to shock on three. One, I'm clear."* (Check to make sure you are clear of contact with the patient, the stretcher, and the equipment.)
- *"Two, you are clear."* (Make a visual check to ensure that no one continues to touch the patient or stretcher. In particular, check the person providing ventilations. That person's hands should not be touching the ventilatory adjuncts, including the endotracheal tube! Be sure oxygen is not flowing across the patient's chest. Turn oxygen off or direct flow away from the patient's chest.)
- *"Three, everybody's clear."* (Check yourself one more time before pressing the "shock" buttons.)

13. Adhesive electrode pads preferred; if paddles used, apply 25 lb pressure on both paddles.
14. Press the "discharge" buttons simultaneously on paddles or the shock button on the unit.
15. Check the monitor. If tachycardia persists, increase the joules according to the electrical cardioversion algorithm.
16. **Reset the sync mode after each synchronized cardioversion because most defibrillators default back to unsynchronized mode.** This default allows an immediate shock if the cardioversion produces VF.

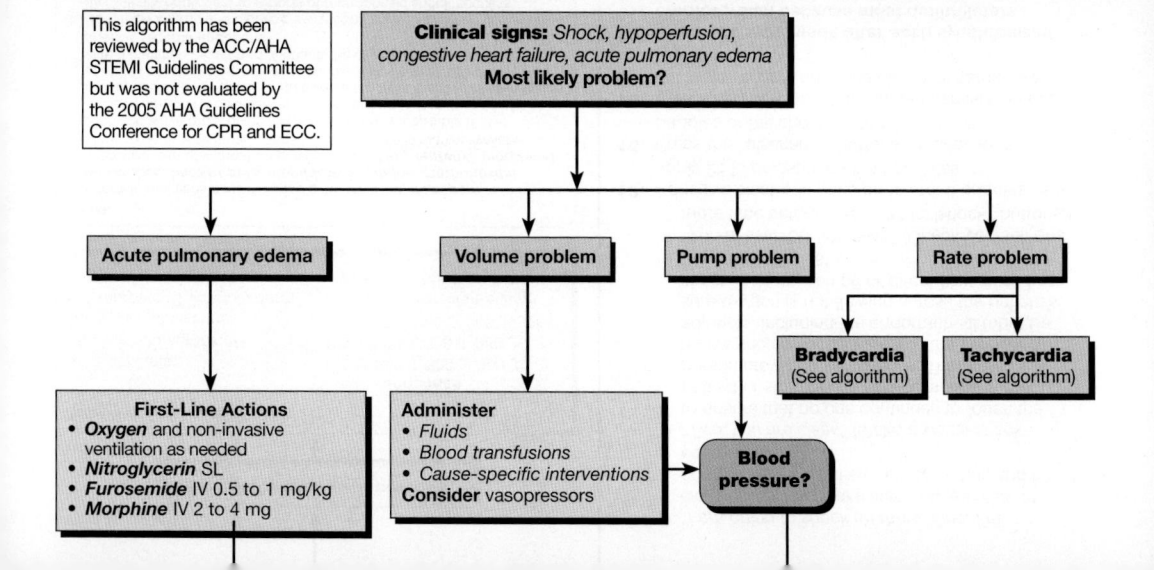

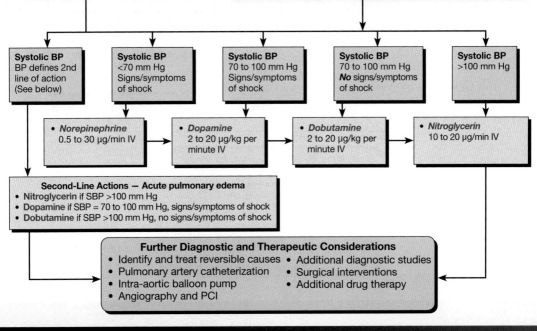

Systolic BP
BP defines 2nd line of action (See below)

Systolic BP
<70 mm Hg
Signs/symptoms of shock

Systolic BP
70 to 100 mm Hg
Signs/symptoms of shock

Systolic BP
70 to 100 mm Hg
No signs/symptoms of shock

Systolic BP
>100 mm Hg

- *Norepinephrine*
0.5 to 30 µg/min IV

- *Dopamine*
2 to 20 µg/kg per minute IV

- *Dobutamine*
2 to 20 µg/kg per minute IV

- *Nitroglycerin*
10 to 20 µg/min IV

Second-Line Actions — Acute pulmonary edema
- Nitroglycerin if SBP >100 mm Hg
- Dopamine if SBP = 70 to 100 mm Hg, signs/symptoms of shock
- Dobutamine if SBP >100 mm Hg, no signs/symptoms of shock

Further Diagnostic and Therapeutic Considerations
- Identify and treat reversible causes
- Pulmonary artery catheterization
- Intra-aortic balloon pump
- Angiography and PCI
- Additional diagnostic studies
- Surgical interventions
- Additional drug therapy

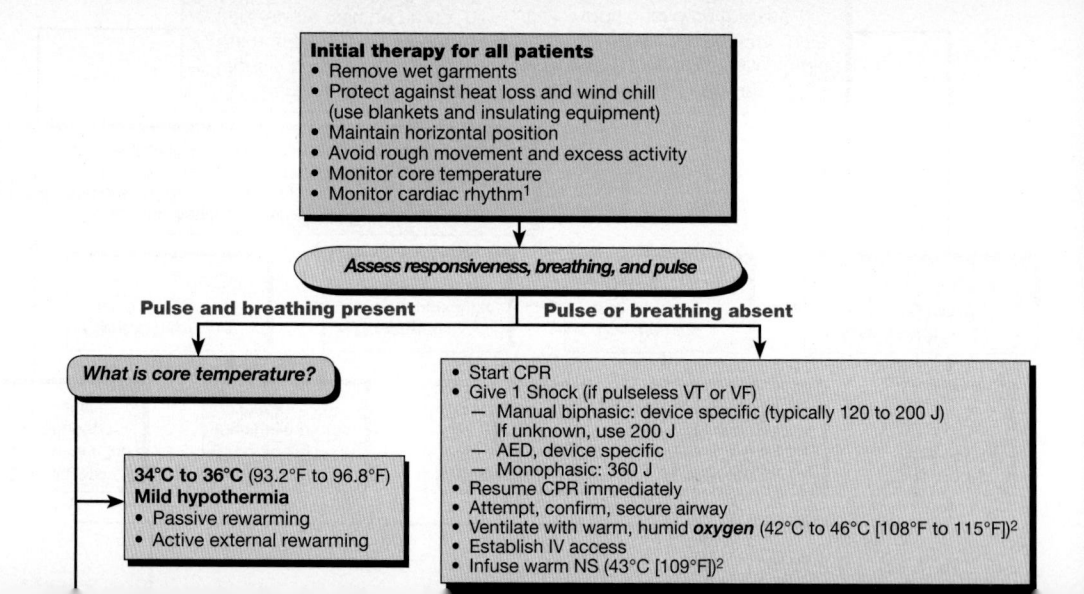

Initial therapy for all patients
- Remove wet garments
- Protect against heat loss and wind chill (use blankets and insulating equipment)
- Maintain horizontal position
- Avoid rough movement and excess activity
- Monitor core temperature
- Monitor cardiac rhythm[1]

Assess responsiveness, breathing, and pulse

Pulse and breathing present

Pulse or breathing absent

What is core temperature?

34°C to 36°C (93.2°F to 96.8°F)
Mild hypothermia
- Passive rewarming
- Active external rewarming

- Start CPR
- Give 1 Shock (if pulseless VT or VF)
  - Manual biphasic: device specific (typically 120 to 200 J) If unknown, use 200 J
  - AED, device specific
  - Monophasic: 360 J
- Resume CPR immediately
- Attempt, confirm, secure airway
- Ventilate with warm, humid ***oxygen*** (42°C to 46°C [108°F to 115°F])[2]
- Establish IV access
- Infuse warm NS (43°C [109°F])[2]

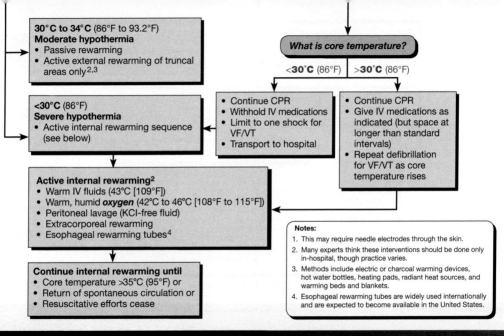

30°C to 34°C (86°F to 93.2°F)
Moderate hypothermia
- Passive rewarming
- Active external rewarming of truncal areas only [2,3]

<30°C (86°F)
Severe hypothermia
- Active internal rewarming sequence (see below)

What is core temperature?

<30°C (86°F)
- Continue CPR
- Withhold IV medications
- Limit to one shock for VF/VT
- Transport to hospital

>30°C (86°F)
- Continue CPR
- Give IV medications as indicated (but space at longer than standard intervals)
- Repeat defibrillation for VF/VT as core temperature rises

Active internal rewarming [2]
- Warm IV fluids (43°C [109°F])
- Warm, humid *oxygen* (42°C to 46°C [108°F to 115°F])
- Peritoneal lavage (KCl-free fluid)
- Extracorporeal rewarming
- Esophageal rewarming tubes [4]

Continue internal rewarming until
- Core temperature >35°C (95°F) or
- Return of spontaneous circulation or
- Resuscitative efforts cease

Notes:
1. This may require needle electrodes through the skin.
2. Many experts think these interventions should be done only in-hospital, though practice varies.
3. Methods include electric or charcoal warming devices, hot water bottles, heating pads, radiant heat sources, and warming beds and blankets.
4. Esophageal rewarming tubes are widely used internationally and are expected to become available in the United States.

Identify signs of possible stroke

Critical EMS assessments and actions
- Support ABCs; give **oxygen** if needed
- Perform prehospital stroke assessment
- Establish time when patient last known normal (*Note:* therapies may be available beyond 3 hours from onset)
- Transport; consider triage to a center with a stroke unit if appropriate; consider bringing a witness, family member, or caregiver
- Alert hospital
- Check glucose if possible

**NINDS
TIME
GOALS**

ED Arrival

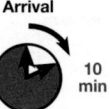

10 min

Immediate general assessment and stabilization
- Assess ABCs, vital signs
- Provide **oxygen** if hypoxemic
- Obtain IV access and blood samples
- Check glucose; treat if indicated
- Perform neurologic screening assessment
- Activate stroke team
- Order emergent CT scan of brain
- Obtain 12-lead ECG

ED Arrival

25 min

Immediate neurologic assessment by stroke team or designee
- Review patient history
- Establish symptom onset
- Perform neurologic examination (NIH Stroke Scale or Canadian Neurologic Scale)

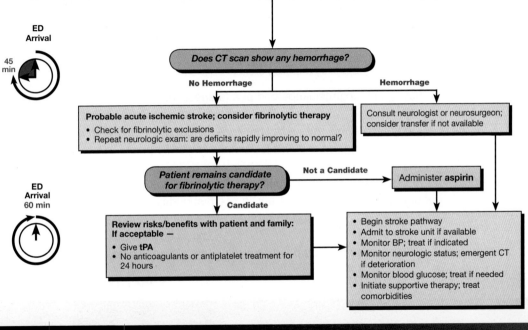

ED Arrival 45 min

Does CT scan show any hemorrhage?

No Hemorrhage

Hemorrhage

Probable acute ischemic stroke; consider fibrinolytic therapy
- Check for fibrinolytic exclusions
- Repeat neurologic exam: are deficits rapidly improving to normal?

Consult neurologist or neurosurgeon; consider transfer if not available

ED Arrival 60 min

Patient remains candidate for fibrinolytic therapy?

Not a Candidate

Administer **aspirin**

Candidate

Review risks/benefits with patient and family: If acceptable —
- Give **tPA**
- No anticoagulants or antiplatelet treatment for 24 hours

- Begin stroke pathway
- Admit to stroke unit if available
- Monitor BP; treat if indicated
- Monitor neurologic status; emergent CT if deterioration
- Monitor blood glucose; treat if needed
- Initiate supportive therapy; treat comorbidities

The 7 D's of Stroke Care

The 7 D's of stroke care highlight the major steps in diagnosis and treatment of stroke and key points at which delays can occur:

- **Detection** of the onset of signs and symptoms of stroke
- **Dispatch** of EMS (by telephoning 911 or the emergency response number)
- **Delivery** with advanced prehospital notification to a hospital capable of providing acute stroke care
- **Door** of the ED, including arrival and urgent triage in the ED
- **Data**, including computed tomography (CT) scan and interpretation of the scan
- **Decision** regarding treatment, including fibrinolytics
- **Drug** administration (as appropriate) and postadministration monitoring

Hazinski M. D-mystifying recognition and management of stroke. *Currents in Emergency Cardiovascular Care.* 1996;7:8.

Out-of-Hospital Assessment of the Patient With Acute Stroke

- Ensure adequate airway
- Measure vital signs frequently
- Conduct general medical/trauma assessment
  - Trauma of head or neck
  - Cardiovascular abnormalities
  - Check pupils
  - Check glucose level
- Conduct neurologic examination
  - Level of consciousness
  - Cincinnati Prehospital Stroke Scale (+/–)
  - Los Angeles Prehospital Stroke Screen (+/–)
  - Glasgow Coma Scale (score/15)
  - Report right and left limb movements
  - Report meningeal signs (yes/no)
  - Report time of onset of symptoms
  - Report any seizure activity
  - Provide prearrival notification to receiving hospital of potential stroke patient

The Cincinnati Prehospital Stroke Scale

(Kothari R, et al. *Acad Emerg Med*. 1997;4:986-990.)

Facial Droop (have the patient show teeth or smile):
- Normal—both sides of face move equally
- Abnormal—one side of face does not move as well as the other side

Arm Drift (patient closes eyes and extends both arms straight out, with palms up, for 10 seconds):
- Normal—both arms move the same *or* both arms do not move at all (other findings, such as pronator drift, may be helpful)
- Abnormal—one arm does not move *or* one arm drifts down compared with the other

Abnormal Speech (have the patient say "you can't teach an old dog new tricks"):
- Normal—patient uses correct words with no slurring
- Abnormal—patient slurs words, uses the wrong words, or is unable to speak

Interpretation: If any *1* of these 3 signs is abnormal, the probability of a stroke is 72%.

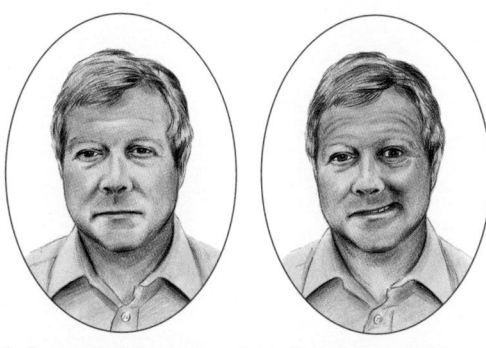

Left: normal. Right: stroke patient with facial droop (right side of face).

Los Angeles Prehospital Stroke Screen (LAPSS)

For *evaluation of acute, noncomatose, nontraumatic neurologic complaint.* If items 1 through 6 are *all* checked "Yes" (or "Unknown"), provide prearrival notification to hospital of potential stroke patient. If any item is checked "No," return to appropriate treatment protocol. *Interpretation:* 93% of patients with stroke will have a positive LAPSS score (sensitivity = 93%), and 97% of those with a positive LAPSS score will have a stroke (specificity = 97%). Note that the patient may still be experiencing a stroke if LAPSS criteria are not met.

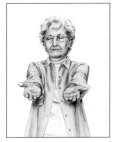

Criteria	Yes	Unknown	No
1. Age >45 years	❑	❑	❑
2. History of seizures or epilepsy **absent**	❑	❑	❑
3. Symptom duration <24 hours	❑	❑	❑
4. At baseline, patient is **not** wheelchair bound or bedridden	❑	❑	❑
5. Blood glucose between 60 and 400 mg/dL	❑	❑	❑

6. *Obvious asymmetry* (right vs left) in *any* of the following 3 exam categories (must be unilateral):

	Equal	R Weak	L Weak
Facial smile/grimace	❑	❑ Droop	❑ Droop
Grip	❑	❑ Weak grip	❑ Weak grip
		❑ No grip	❑ No grip
Arm strength	❑	❑ Drifts down	❑ Drifts down
		❑ Falls rapidly	❑ Falls rapidly

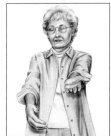

One-sided motor weakness (right arm).

Kidwell CS, Saver JL, Schubert GB, Eckstein M, Starkman S. Design and retrospective analysis of the Los Angeles prehospital stroke screen (LAPSS). *Prehosp Emerg Care.* 1998;2:267-273.

Kidwell CS, Starkman S, Eckstein M, Weems K, Saver JL. Identifying stroke in the field: prospective validation of the Los Angeles Prehospital Stroke Screen (LAPSS). *Stroke.* 2000;31:71-76.

Glasgow Coma Scale

	Score (maximum = 15)
Eye opening	
Spontaneous	4
In response to speech	3
In response to pain	2
None	1
Best verbal response	
Oriented conversation	5
Confused conversation	4
Inappropriate words	3
Incomprehensible sounds	2
None	1
Best motor response	
Obeys	6
Localizes	5
Withdraws	4
Abnormal flexion	3
Abnormal extension	2
None	1

Interpretation:
Score 14 to 15: Mild dysfunction
Score 11 to 13: Moderate to severe dysfunction
Score 10: Severe dysfunction

Hunt and Hess Scale for Subarachnoid Hemorrhage

Grade	Neurologic Status
1	Asymptomatic
2	Severe headache or nuchal rigidity; no neurologic deficit
3	Drowsy; minimal neurologic deficit
4	Stuporous; moderate to severe hemiparesis
5	Deep coma; decerebrate posturing

General Management of the Acute Stroke Patient

1. **Intravenous fluids:** Avoid D_5W and excessive fluid loading.

2. **Blood sugar:** Determine immediately. Bolus of 50% dextrose if hypoglycemic; insulin if >140-185 mg/dL (>7.8-10.3 mmol/L).

3. **Thiamine:** 100 mg if malnourished, alcoholic.

4. **Oxygen:** Pulse oximetry. Supplement for oxygen saturation <92%.

5. **Acetaminophen:** If febrile.

6. **NPO:** If at risk for aspiration.

General Brain-Oriented Intensive Care

- Normotension throughout coma (eg, mean arterial pressure 90 to 100 mm Hg or normal systolic level for patient): titrate fluids and vasoactive agents as needed.
- Adequate ventilation (arterial P_{CO_2} about 35 mm Hg).
- Maintain adequate oxygen saturation (≥92%); use lowest positive end-expiratory pressure possible.
- Arterial pH 7.3 to 7.5.
- Immobilization (neuromuscular paralysis) as needed.
- Sedation (eg, morphine or diazepam) as needed.
- Anticonvulsants (eg, diazepam, phenytoin, or barbiturates) as needed.
- Normalization of blood chemistry (hematocrit, electrolytes, osmolality, and glucose). Bolus glucose if hypoglycemic; administer insulin if glucose >140-185 mg/dL (>7.8-10.3 mmol/L).
- Administer thiamine (100 mg) if malnourished, alcoholic.
- Osmotherapy (mannitol or glycerol) as needed for monitored intracranial pressure elevation or secondary neurologic deterioration.
- Avoid administration of hypotonic fluids, maintain serum sodium concentration, avoid excessive fluid loading.
- Begin treatment for temperature >37.5°C.
- Nutritional support started by 48 hours.

All boxes must be checked before tPA can be given.
Note: The following checklist includes FDA-approved indications and contraindications for tPA administration for acute ischemic stroke. A physician with expertise in acute stroke care may modify this list.

Inclusion Criteria *(all **Yes** boxes in this section must be checked):*
Yes

☐ Age 18 years or older?
☐ Clinical diagnosis of ischemic stroke with a measurable neurologic deficit?
☐ Time of symptom onset (when patient was last seen normal) well established as <180 minutes (3 hours) before treatment would begin?

Exclusion Criteria *(all **No** boxes in "Contraindications" section must be checked):*
Contraindications:

No

☐ Evidence of intracranial hemorrhage on pretreatment noncontrast head CT?
☐ Clinical presentation suggestive of subarachnoid hemorrhage even with normal CT?
☐ CT shows multilobar infarction (hypodensity greater than one third cerebral hemisphere)?
☐ History of intracranial hemorrhage?
☐ Uncontrolled hypertension: At the time treatment should begin, systolic pressure remains >185 mm Hg or diastolic pressure remains >110 mm Hg despite repeated measurements?
☐ Known arteriovenous malformation, neoplasm, or aneurysm?
☐ Seizure with post-ictal residual neurologic impairment? *Note:* Seizure alone at time of onset is not an absolute contraindication.

- ❏ Active internal bleeding or acute trauma (fracture)?
- ❏ Acute bleeding diathesis, including but not limited to
  - Platelet count <100 000/mm^3?
  - Heparin received within 48 hours, resulting in an activated partial thromboplastin time (aPTT) that is greater than upper limit of normal for laboratory?
  - Current use of anticoagulant (eg, warfarin sodium) that has produced an elevated international normalized ratio (INR) >1.7 or prothrombin time (PT) >15 seconds?*
- ❏ Within 3 months of intracranial or intraspinal surgery, serious head trauma, or previous stroke?
- ❏ Arterial puncture at a noncompressible site within past 7 days?

Relative Contraindications/Precautions:

Recent experience suggests that under some circumstances—with careful consideration and weighing of risk-to-benefit ratio—patients may receive fibrinolytic therapy despite one or more relative contraindications. Consider the pros and cons of tPA administration carefully if any of these relative contraindications is present:

- Only minor or rapidly improving stroke symptoms (clearing spontaneously)
- Within 14 days of major surgery or serious trauma
- Recent gastrointestinal or urinary tract hemorrhage (within previous 21 days)
- Recent acute myocardial infarction (within previous 3 months)
- Postmyocardial infarction pericarditis
- Abnormal blood glucose level (<50 or >400 mg/dL [<2.8 or >22.2 mmol/L])

*In patients without recent use of oral anticoagulants or heparin, treatment with tPA can be initiated before availability of coagulation study results but should be discontinued if the INR is >1.7 or the partial thromboplastin time is elevated by local laboratory standards.

Blood Pressure Level mm Hg	Treatment
A. For patients who are not eligible for fibrinolytic therapy	
Systolic ≤220 or diastolic ≤120	• Observe unless other end-organ involvement (eg, aortic dissection, acute myocardial infarction, pulmonary edema, hypertensive encephalopathy). Withhold emergency anti-hypertensive agents unless the systolic BP is >220 mm Hg or mean BP is >120 mm Hg. • Treat other symptoms of stroke (eg, headache, pain, agitation, nausea, vomiting). • Treat other acute complications of stroke, including hypoxia, increased intracranial pressure, seizures, or hypoglycemia.
Systolic >220 or diastolic 121 to 140	• Labetalol 10 to 20 mg IV over 1 to 2 minutes. • May repeat or double every 10 minutes (max dose 300 mg) **or** • Nicardipine 5 mg/h IV infusion as initial dose; titrate to desired effect by increasing 2.5 mg/h every 5 minutes to max of 15 mg/h. • Aim for a 15% to 25% reduction in BP within first 24 hours.
Diastolic >140	• Nitroprusside 0.5 µg/kg per minute IV infusion as initial dose with continuous blood pressure monitoring. • Aim for a 15% to 25% reduction in BP within first 24 hours.

B. For patients who are otherwise eligible for fibrinolytic therapy	
Pretreatment	
Systolic >185 or diastolic >110	• Labetalol 10 to 20 mg IV over 1 to 2 minutes, may repeat × 1 **or**
	• Nitropaste 1 to 2 inches **or**
	• Nicardipine infusion, 5 mg/h, titrate up by 2.5 mg/h q 5 to 15 minutes, max dose 15 mg/h; when desired BP is attained, reduce to 3 mg/h.
	• If BP remains >185/110 mm Hg, do not administer tPA.
During/after treatment	
Monitor blood pressure	• Check BP every 15 minutes during therapy and for 2 hours after therapy; then every 30 minutes for 6 hours, and then every hour for 16 hours.
Systolic >230 or diastolic 121 to 140	• Labetalol 10 mg IV over 1 to 2 minutes, may repeat every 10 to 20 minutes (max dose 300 mg) **or**
	• Labetalol 10 mg IV followed by an infusion of 2 to 8 mg/min **or**
	• Nicardipine 5 mg/h IV infusion as initial dose and titrate to desired effect by increasing 2.5 mg/h every 5 minutes to maximum of 15 mg/h; **or**
	• If BP is not controlled by either labetalol or nicardipine, consider sodium nitroprusside.
Systolic 180 to 230 or diastolic 105 to 120	• Labetalol 10 mg IV over 1 to 2 minutes, may repeat every 10 to 20 minutes (max dose 300 mg) **or**
	• Labetalol 10 mg IV followed by an infusion at 2 to 8 mg/min.

This section contains recommendations consistent with the ACC/AHA 2007 Guideline Update for the Management of Patients With Unstable Angina and Non–ST-Segment Elevation Myocardial Infarction. Jeffrey Anderson, MD, FACC, FAHA, chair, and the ACC/AHA Guideline for the Management of Patients With ST-Segment Elevation Myocardial Infarction, 2007 Focused Update. Elliott M Antman, MD, FACC, FAHA, chair, and consistent with the 2005 AHA Guidelines for CPR and ECC.

Natural History of Coronary Artery Disease: Evolution to the Major Acute Coronary Syndromes

Early plaque formation

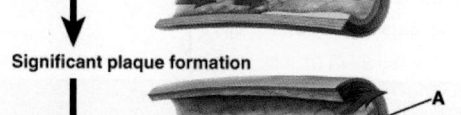

Significant plaque formation

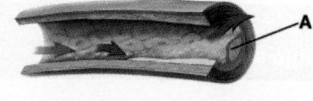

Acute Coronary Syndromes. Patients with coronary atherosclerosis may develop a spectrum of clinical syndromes representing varying degrees of coronary artery occlusion. These syndromes include unstable angina, non–ST-segment elevation MI (NSTEMI), and ST-segment elevation MI (STEMI). Sudden cardiac death may occur with each syndrome.

A Unstable plaque
Disruption (rupture/erosion) of a lipid-laden plaque with a thin cap is the usual cause of an ACS. The majority of these plaques are not hemodynamically significant before rupture. An inflammatory component in the subendothelial area further weakens and predisposes the plaque to rupture. Speed of blood flow, turbulence, and vessel anatomy may also be important contributing factors. Other causes occur in a minority of patients and include spasm, coronary embolism, and spontaneous dissection.

B Plaque rupture/erosion
After rupture or erosion a monolayer of platelets covers the surface of the ruptured plaque (platelet adhesion). The active plaque and platelets attract and activate additional platelets (platelet aggregation). Fibrinogen cross-links platelets, and the coagulation system is activated with thrombin generation.

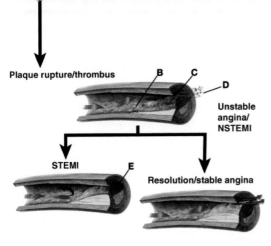

Plaque rupture/thrombus

Unstable angina/NSTEMI

STEMI

Resolution/stable angina

C Unstable angina
A partially occluding thrombus produces symptoms of ischemia, which are prolonged and may occur at rest. At this stage the thrombus is platelet-rich. Therapy with antiplatelet agents such as aspirin, clopidogrel, and GP IIb/IIIa receptor inhibitors is most effective at this time. Fibrinolytic therapy is *not* effective and may paradoxically accelerate occlusion by the release of clot-bound thrombin, which promotes coagulation. An intermittently occlusive thrombus or clot microemboli may cause myocardial necrosis, producing an NSTEMI.

D Microemboli
As the clot enlarges, microemboli may originate from the thrombus and lodge in the coronary microvasculature, causing small elevations of cardiac troponins. These patients are at highest risk for progression to STEMI or Major Adverse Cardiac Events (MACE).

E Occlusive thrombus
If the thrombus occludes the coronary vessel for a prolonged period, a STEMI usually occurs. This clot is rich in thrombin; early/prompt fibrinolysis or primary percutaneous coronary intervention (PCI) may limit infarct size and complications of MI (if performed sufficiently early).

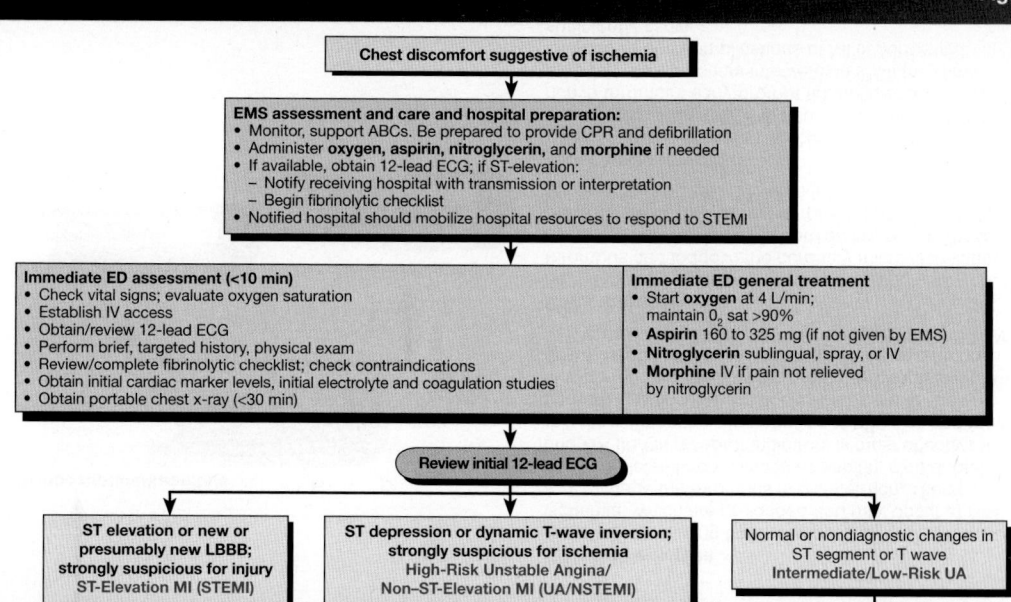

Chest discomfort suggestive of ischemia

EMS assessment and care and hospital preparation:
- Monitor, support ABCs. Be prepared to provide CPR and defibrillation
- Administer **oxygen, aspirin, nitroglycerin,** and **morphine** if needed
- If available, obtain 12-lead ECG; if ST-elevation:
  – Notify receiving hospital with transmission or interpretation
  – Begin fibrinolytic checklist
- Notified hospital should mobilize hospital resources to respond to STEMI

Immediate ED assessment (<10 min)
- Check vital signs; evaluate oxygen saturation
- Establish IV access
- Obtain/review 12-lead ECG
- Perform brief, targeted history, physical exam
- Review/complete fibrinolytic checklist; check contraindications
- Obtain initial cardiac marker levels, initial electrolyte and coagulation studies
- Obtain portable chest x-ray (<30 min)

Immediate ED general treatment
- Start **oxygen** at 4 L/min; maintain O_2 sat >90%
- **Aspirin** 160 to 325 mg (if not given by EMS)
- **Nitroglycerin** sublingual, spray, or IV
- **Morphine** IV if pain not relieved by nitroglycerin

Review initial 12-lead ECG

ST elevation or new or presumably new LBBB; strongly suspicious for injury
ST-Elevation MI (STEMI)

ST depression or dynamic T-wave inversion; strongly suspicious for ischemia
High-Risk Unstable Angina/Non–ST-Elevation MI (UA/NSTEMI)

Normal or nondiagnostic changes in ST segment or T wave
Intermediate/Low-Risk UA

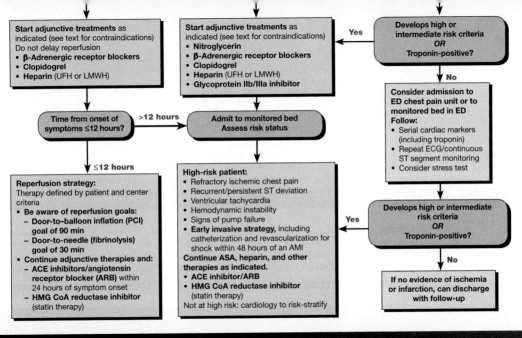

Start adjunctive treatments as indicated (see text for contraindications)
Do not delay reperfusion
- β-Adrenergic receptor blockers
- Clopidogrel
- Heparin (UFH or LMWH)

Start adjunctive treatments as indicated (see text for contraindications)
- Nitroglycerin
- β-Adrenergic receptor blockers
- Clopidogrel
- Heparin (UFH or LMWH)
- Glycoprotein IIb/IIIa inhibitor

Yes ← Develops high or intermediate risk criteria *OR* Troponin-positive?

No ↓

Consider admission to ED chest pain unit or to monitored bed in ED
Follow:
- Serial cardiac markers (including troponin)
- Repeat ECG/continuous ST segment monitoring
- Consider stress test

Time from onset of symptoms ≤12 hours? **>12 hours** → Admit to monitored bed Assess risk status

≤12 hours ↓

Reperfusion strategy:
Therapy defined by patient and center criteria
- Be aware of reperfusion goals:
  - Door-to–balloon inflation (PCI) goal of 90 min
  - Door-to-needle (fibrinolysis) goal of 30 min
- Continue adjunctive therapies and:
  - ACE inhibitors/angiotensin receptor blocker (ARB) within 24 hours of symptom onset
  - HMG CoA reductase inhibitor (statin therapy)

High-risk patient:
- Refractory ischemic chest pain
- Recurrent/persistent ST deviation
- Ventricular tachycardia
- Hemodynamic instability
- Signs of pump failure
- **Early invasive strategy**, including catheterization and revascularization for shock within 48 hours of an AMI
Continue ASA, heparin, and other therapies as indicated.
- ACE inhibitor/ARB
- HMG CoA reductase inhibitor (statin therapy)
Not at high risk: cardiology to risk-stratify

Yes ← Develops high or intermediate risk criteria *OR* Troponin-positive?

No ↓

If no evidence of ischemia or infarction, can discharge with follow-up

Likelihood That Signs and Symptoms Represent an ACS Secondary to CAD

Patients should undergo risk assessment that focuses on history, physical findings, ECG results, and biomarkers. Results should be considered in patient management. Table modified from Braunwald et al. ACC/AHA Guidelines for the Management of Patients With Unstable Angina and Non–ST-Segment Elevation Myocardial Infarction: Executive Summary and Recommendations. *Circulation.* 2000;102:1193-1209.

Part I. Chest Pain Patients Without ST-Segment Elevation: Likelihood of Ischemic Etiology			
	A. High likelihood High likelihood that chest pain is of ischemic etiology if patient has *any* of the findings in the column below:	**B. Intermediate likelihood** Intermediate likelihood that chest pain is of ischemic etiology if patient has NO findings in column A and *any* of the findings in the column below:	**C. Low likelihood** Low likelihood that chest pain is of ischemic etiology if patient has **NO** findings in column **A or B**. Patients may have any of the findings in the column below:
History	■ Chief symptom is chest or left arm discomfort *plus* — Current discomfort reproduces symptoms of prior documented angina — Known CAD, MI	■ Chief symptom is chest or left arm pain or discomfort ■ Age >70 years ■ Male sex ■ Diabetes mellitus	■ Probable ischemic symptoms ■ Recent cocaine use

Physical exam	■ Transient mitral regurgitation ■ Hypotension ■ Diaphoresis ■ Pulmonary edema or rales	■ Extracardiac vascular disease	■ Chest discomfort reproduced by palpation
ECG	■ New (or presumed new) transient ST deviation (≥0.5 mm) *or* T-wave inversion (≥2 mm) with symptoms	■ Fixed Q waves ■ ST depression 0.5 to 1 mm or T-wave inversion >1 mm	■ Normal ECG *or* T-wave flattening *or* T-wave inversion <1 mm in leads with dominant R waves
Cardiac markers	■ Elevated troponin I or T ■ Elevated CK-MB	■ Normal	■ Normal

High (A) or Intermediate (B) Likelihood of Ischemia

(continued on next page)

(continued from previous page)

▼

Part II. Risk of Death or Nonfatal MI Over the Short Term in Patients With Chest Pain With High or Intermediate Likelihood of Ischemia (Columns A and B in Part I)

	High risk: Risk is high if patient has *any* of the following findings:	Intermediate risk: Risk is intermediate if patient has *any* of the following findings:	Low risk: Risk is low if patient has NO high- or intermediate-risk features; may have any of the following:
History	■ Accelerating tempo of ischemic symptoms over prior 48 hours	■ Prior MI *or* ■ Peripheral-artery disease *or* ■ Cerebrovascular disease *or* ■ CABG, prior aspirin use	
Character of Pain	■ Prolonged, continuing (>20 min) rest pain	■ Prolonged (>20 min) rest angina is now resolved (moderate to high likelihood of CAD) ■ Rest angina (≤20 min) or relieved by rest or sublingual nitrate ■ Nocturnal angina	■ Increased angina, frequency, severity, or duration ■ Angina provoked at lower threshold

		New-onset functional angina (Class III or IV) in past 2 weeks without prolonged rest pain (but with moderate or high likelihood of CAD [see Part I])	New-onset angina with onset 2 weeks to 2 months prior to presentation
Physical findings	■ Pulmonary edema secondary to ischemia ■ New or worse mitral regurgitation murmur ■ Hypotension, bradycardia, tachycardia ■ S_3 gallop or new or worsening rales ■ Age >75 years	■ Age >70 years	
ECG	■ Transient ST-segment deviation (≥0.5 mm) with rest angina ■ New or presumably new bundle branch block ■ Sustained VT	■ T-wave changes ■ Pathologic Q waves or resting ST-depression (<1 mm) in multiple lead groups (anterior, inferior, lateral)	■ Normal or unchanged ECG during an episode of chest discomfort
Cardiac markers	■ Elevated cardiac troponin I or T (CDL)* ■ Elevated CK-MB	Any of the above findings PLUS ■ Result between CDL and MDL.*	■ Normal

*Providers should be familiar with the specific troponin assay used by their clinical laboratory. The clinical decision limit (CDL) is the value determined to represent an abnormal elevation, diagnostic of MI. Often referred to as a "positive result." The minimal detectable limit (MDL) is the lowest value that can be detected by the specific troponin test. These values are often called "grey zone" values (or possibly "weakly positive").

Initial Management in the Field and Emergency Department

Immediate Assessment

- Vital signs, including blood pressure
- Oxygen saturation
- IV access
- 12-lead ECG
- Brief, targeted history and physical exam (to identify reperfusion candidates)
- Fibrinolytic checklist; check contraindications
- Obtain initial cardiac markers
- Initial electrolyte and coagulation studies
- Portable chest x-ray <30 minutes
- Assess for the following:
  - Heart rate ≥100/min and SBP ≤100 mm Hg *or*
  - Pulmonary edema (rales) *or*
  - Signs of shock

  If any of these conditions is present, consider triage to a facility capable of cardiac catheterization and revascularization.

Out-of-Hospital Fibrinolytic Therapy for STEMI

- When EMS has capability, fibrinolysis should be started within 30 minutes of EMS arrival.
- EMS assessment (12-lead ECG and chest pain checklist in field), triage, and prearrival notification reduce time to in-hospital fibrinolytics.
- Prehospital fibrinolytic therapy is recommended only in systems with established protocols and checklists, experience in ACLS, ability to communicate with receiving institution and medical director with training/experience in the management of STEMI.

Fibrinolytic Checklist for STEMI

- A prehospital fibrinolytic checklist in the absence of the cabability to administer fibrinolytic therapy is useful to identify patients for triage to a PCI destination hospital when available.

Early Recognition and Access, EMS Response, and Medical Systems Goals

Early Recognition and Access
- Most treatment delay is due to patient denial. Physicians should educate patients and families about the signs and symptoms of ACS and the importance of early EMS activation. Patients with known coronary disease often delay longer.
- EMS transport is better than family transport.

Medical System Goals: EMS Transport (Recommended)
- If EMS has fibrinolytic capability and the patient qualifies for therapy, out-of-hospital fibrinolysis should be started within 30 minutes of arrival of EMS on the scene.
- If EMS is not capable of administering out-of-hospital fibrinolysis and the patient is transported to a *non*–PCI-capable hospital, the door-to-needle time should be within 30 minutes when fibrinolysis is indicated.
- If EMS is not capable of administering out-of-hospital fibrinolysis and the patient is transported to a PCI-capable hospital, the EMS arrival-to-balloon time should be within 90 minutes.
- If EMS takes the patient to a *non*–PCI-capable hospital, it is appropriate to consider emergency *interhospital transfer* of the patient to a PCI-capable hospital for mechanical revascularization if
  - There is a contraindication to fibrinolysis.
  - PCI can be initiated promptly (≤90 minutes from first medical contact–to-balloon time) at the PCI-capable hospital.
  - Fibrinolysis is administered and is unsuccessful (ie, "rescue PCI").
- It is reasonable that patients with STEMI who are at especially high risk of dying, including those with severe congestive heart failure (CHF), be considered for immediate or prompt secondary transfer (ie, primary-receiving hospital door-to-departure time less than 30 minutes) to facilities capable of cardiac catheterization and rapid revascularization.

Out-of-Hospital ECG
EMS responders should be trained and equipped to obtain 12-lead ECGs. An out-of-hospital 12-lead ECG and advance notification of the ED can reduce time to reperfusion.
- Reduces time to fibrinolytic therapy and coronary angiography/PCI.
- Allows triage of patients in shock with STEMI to interventional facilities.

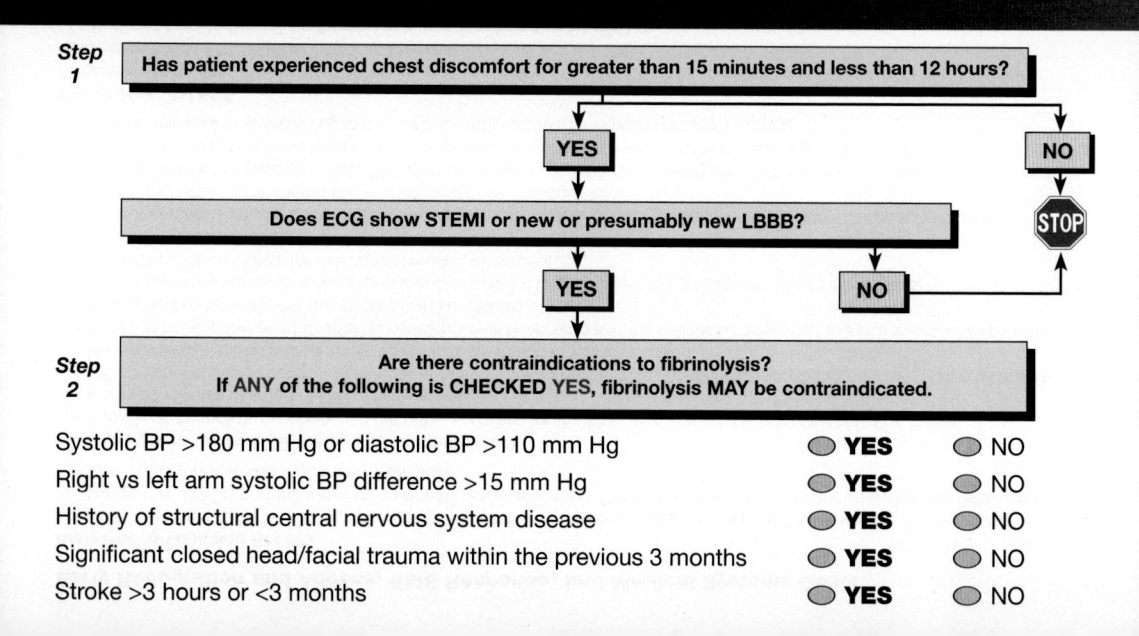

The Acute Coronary Syndromes: Fibrinolytic Checklist for STEMI

ACLS

Step 1

Has patient experienced chest discomfort for greater than 15 minutes and less than 12 hours?

YES → NO → STOP

Does ECG show STEMI or new or presumably new LBBB?

YES → NO →

Step 2

Are there contraindications to fibrinolysis?
If ANY of the following is CHECKED YES, fibrinolysis MAY be contraindicated.

Systolic BP >180 mm Hg or diastolic BP >110 mm Hg	YES	NO
Right vs left arm systolic BP difference >15 mm Hg	YES	NO
History of structural central nervous system disease	YES	NO
Significant closed head/facial trauma within the previous 3 months	YES	NO
Stroke >3 hours or <3 months	YES	NO

Recent (within 6 weeks) major trauma, surgery (including laser eye surgery), GI/GU bleed	◯ **YES**	◯ NO
Any history of intracranial hemorrhage	◯ **YES**	◯ NO
Bleeding or clotting problem on blood thinners	◯ **YES**	◯ NO
CPR >10 minutes	◯ **YES**	◯ NO
Pregnant female	◯ **YES**	◯ NO
Serious systemic disease (eg, advanced cancer, severe liver or kidney disease)	◯ **YES**	◯ NO

Step 3

> **Is patient at high risk?**
> If ANY of the following is CHECKED YES, consider transfer to PCI facility.

Heart rate ≥100/min AND systolic BP <100 mm Hg	◯ **YES**	◯ NO
Pulmonary edema (rales)	◯ **YES**	◯ NO
Signs of shock (cool, clammy)	◯ **YES**	◯ NO
Contraindications to fibrinolytic therapy	◯ **YES**∗	◯ NO

∗Consider transport to primary PCI facility as destination hospital.

Immediate General Treatment
- Aspirin
- Oxygen
- Nitroglycerin
- Morphine (if unresponsive to nitrates)

Oxygen
Rationale: May limit ischemic myocardial injury, reducing the amount of ST-segment elevation. Its effects on morbidity and mortality in acute infarction are unknown.

Recommendations: 4 L/min per nasal cannula
- **Uncomplicated MI:** Probably not helpful beyond 6 hours.
- **Complicated MI:** (overt pulmonary congestion, Sao_2 <90%): Administer supplementary O_2 at 4 L/min by nasal cannula, titrate as needed. Continue until the patient is stable or hypoxemia is corrected.

Aspirin
Rationale: Inhibits thromboxane A_2 platelet aggregation to reduce coronary reocclusion and recurrent events after fibrinolytic therapy. Also effective for unstable angina.

Recommendations
- For all patients with ACS unless true aspirin allergy (then consider clopidogrel) in either out-of-hospital or ED setting (Class I).
- Give 160 to 325 mg nonenteric-coated orally, crushed or chewed (use rectal suppositories if nausea, vomiting, or active peptic ulcer disease).

Cautions, Contraindications
- Active peptic ulcer disease (use rectal suppositories)
- History of true aspirin allergy
- Bleeding disorders, severe hepatic disease

Nitroglycerin

Rationale: Dilates coronary arteries (particularly in region of plaque disruption) and vascular smooth muscle in veins, arteries, and arterioles. Reduces ischemic pain but is not a substitute for narcotic analgesia.

Recommendations

- Administer to all patients with ACS and ongoing ischemic pain without contraindications.
- Use short-acting nitroglycerin. Route of therapy determined by patient condition. Typically IV therapy (when indicated) is used for patients with AMI to allow precise control of dose. Use SL or spray form in pre-hospital setting or for stable patients.
- IV therapy indicated in the following clinical situations:
  — Ongoing ischemic chest discomfort
  — Management of hypertension
  — Management of pulmonary congestion
- Use for 24 to 48 hours for patients with AMI and CHF, large anterior wall infarction, persistent or recurrent ischemia, or hypertension.
- Continue use (beyond 48 hours) for patients with recurrent angina or persistent pulmonary congestion (nitrate-free interval recommended).

Initial Dose, Route

- SL: 0.3 to 0.4 mg, repeat × 2 at 3- to 5-minute intervals **OR**
- Spray: 1 or 2 sprays, may repeat × 2 at 3- to 5-minute intervals **OR**
- IV: 12.5 to 25 µg bolus (if no SL or spray given); then 10 µg/min infusion, titrated (increased at a rate of 10 µg/min every 3 to 5 minutes until symptom response or target arterial pressure is achieved). Ceiling dose of 200 µg/min commonly used.

Treatment Goals

- Relief of ischemic discomfort.
- Systolic blood pressure (SBP) should generally not be reduced to less than 110 mm Hg in previously normotensive patients or to more than 25% below starting mean arterial pressure if hypertension was present.

Cautions, Contraindications

- Contraindicated if SBP <90 mm Hg. Use with caution if at all for borderline hypotension (SBP 90 to 100 mm Hg).
- Contraindicated for severe bradycardia (heart rate <50/min) or tachycardia (>100/min). Use with caution if at all for borderline bradycardia (HR <60/min).
- Use extreme caution in patients who may have RV infarction.
- Contraindicated in patients who have used phospho-diesterase inhibitor for erectile dysfunction (eg, sildenafil and vardenafil within 24 hours; tadalafil within 48 hours).

The Acute Coronary Syndromes: Initial Management

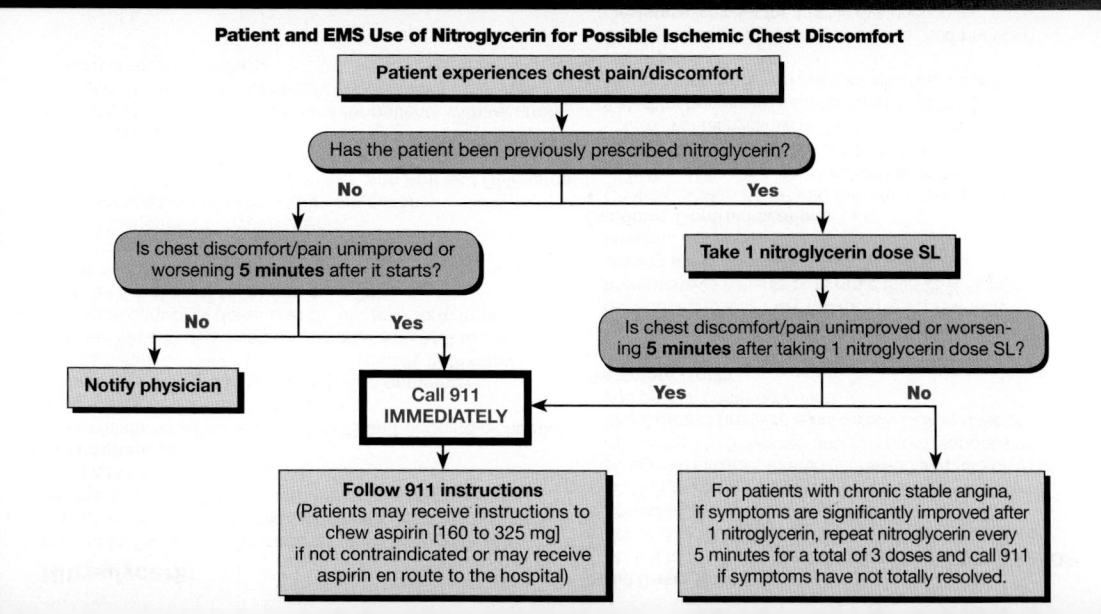

Patient and EMS Use of Nitroglycerin for Possible Ischemic Chest Discomfort

Patient experiences chest pain/discomfort

↓

Has the patient been previously prescribed nitroglycerin?

No / **Yes**

No →

Is chest discomfort/pain unimproved or worsening **5 minutes** after it starts?

No → **Notify physician**

Yes → Call 911 IMMEDIATELY

Yes → **Take 1 nitroglycerin dose SL**

↓

Is chest discomfort/pain unimproved or worsening **5 minutes** after taking 1 nitroglycerin dose SL?

Yes → Call 911 IMMEDIATELY

No →

Call 911 IMMEDIATELY

↓

Follow 911 instructions
(Patients may receive instructions to chew aspirin [160 to 325 mg] if not contraindicated or may receive aspirin en route to the hospital)

For patients with chronic stable angina, if symptoms are significantly improved after 1 nitroglycerin, repeat nitroglycerin every 5 minutes for a total of 3 doses and call 911 if symptoms have not totally resolved.

Morphine

Rationale: Dilates arteries and veins, which redistributes blood volume and reduces ventricular preload and afterload. Decreases oxygen requirements. Can reduce pulmonary edema. Analgesic effects reduce chest pain.

- Indicated for patients with ischemic pain not relieved by nitroglycerin and patients with ACS but no hypotension.
- May be useful to redistribute blood volume in patients with pulmonary edema.

Cautions, Contraindications, and Possible Complications

- Do not use in patients with hypotension or suspected hypovolemia.
- If hypotension develops without pulmonary congestion, administer 200 to 500 mL bolus of NS.

2007 Recommended Dosing

STEMI: Morphine is analgesic of choice (Class I). Give 2 to 4 mg IV; may give additional doses of 2 to 8 mg IV at 5- to 15-minute intervals.

UA/NSTEMI: Give 1 to 5 mg IV only if symptoms are not relieved by nitrates or if symptoms recur. Note: Morphine reduced to Class IIa after safety concern raised by large observational registry showing higher adjusted likelihood of death when morphine was given.

Triage and Assessment of Cardiac Risk in the Emergency Department
Stratifying Patients With Possible or Probable ACS in the ED

- **Protocols must be in place to stratify** chest pain patients by risk of ACS. **The 12-lead ECG is central to ED triage of patients with ACS.** Stratify patients into one of the following subgroups (also see next page):

  1. *ST-segment elevation or new LBBB:* High specificity for evolving STEMI; assess reperfusion eligibility

  2. *ST-segment depression:* Consistent with/strongly suggestive of ischemia; defines a high-risk subset of patients with unstable angina/NSTEMI

  3. *Nondiagnostic or normal ECG:* Further assessment usually needed; evaluation protocols should include repeat ECG or continuous ST-segment monitoring. Serial cardiac markers, myocardial imaging, or 2D echocardiogram may be useful during medical observation in selected patients.

- Clinicians should carefully consider the diagnosis of ACS even in the absence of typical chest discomfort. Consider ACS in patients with

  — Anginal equivalent symptoms, such as dyspnea (LV dysfunction); palpitations, presyncope, and syncope (ischemic ventricular arrhythmias)
  — Atypical left precordial pain or complaint of indigestion or dyspepsia
  — Atypical pain in the elderly, women, and persons with diabetes

- Continually consider other causes of chest pain: aortic dissection, peri-/myocarditis, pulmonary embolus

- **Fibrinolytic therapy:** Administer as soon as possible, optimal door-to-drug time of ≤30 minutes

- **PCI:** Identify reperfusion candidates promptly and achieve balloon inflation as soon as possible with primary PCI, door-to–balloon inflation time of ≤90 minutes

Emergency Department

Triage Recommendations

Symptoms and Signs Requiring Immediate Assessment and ECG Within 10 Minutes of Presentation

- **Chest or epigastric discomfort, nontraumatic in origin with components typical for ischemia or MI**
  - Central substernal compression or crushing pain; pressure, tightness, heaviness, cramping, burning, aching sensation; unexplained indigestion, belching, epigastric pain; radiating pain in neck, jaws, shoulders, back, or 1 or both arms
  - Associated dyspnea, nausea or vomiting, diaphoresis
- **For all patients with ischemic-type chest pain, provide supplementary oxygen, IV access, and continuous ECG monitoring**
- **Prompt interpretation of 12-lead ECG by physician responsible for ACS triage**
- **Initiate protocol for reperfusion therapy for ST-segment elevation MI (STEMI)**
  - Rule out contraindications and assess risk-benefit ratio
  - Consider primary PCI if available or patient is ineligible for fibrinolytics
  - Angiography for cardiogenic shock (PCI or CABG if indicated)
- **Prompt aspirin (160 to 325 mg) if not already administered by EMS or patient**
- **Clopidogrel (300 mg loading dose) for fibrinolytic strategy or reperfusion for ineligible patients**
- **Oral β-blockers for all patients without contraindications. IV β-blockers for hypertensive patients without contraindications**
- **IV nitroglycerin for initial 24 to 48 hours only in patients with AMI and CHF, large anterior infarction, recurrent or persistent ischemia, or hypertension**

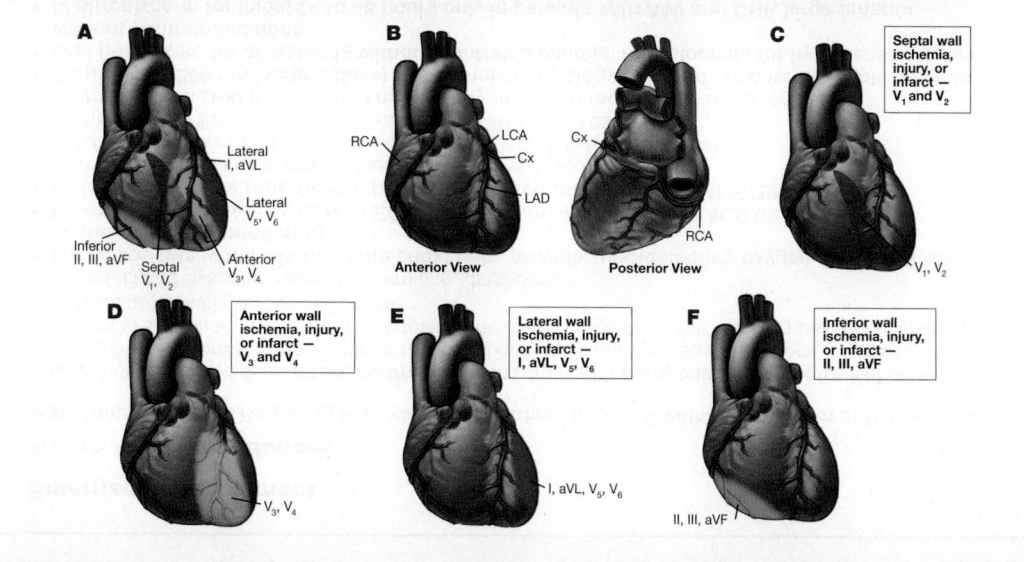

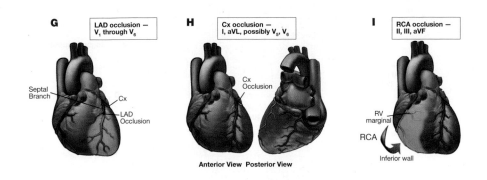

I lateral	aVR	V₁ septal	V₄ anterior
II inferior	aVL lateral	V₂ septal	V₅ lateral
III inferior	aVF inferior	V₃ anterior	V₆ lateral

Localizing ischemia, injury, or infarct using the 12-lead ECG: relationship to coronary artery anatomy.

How to measure ST-segment deviation. A, Inferior MI. ST segment has no low point (it is coved or concave). B, Anterior MI.

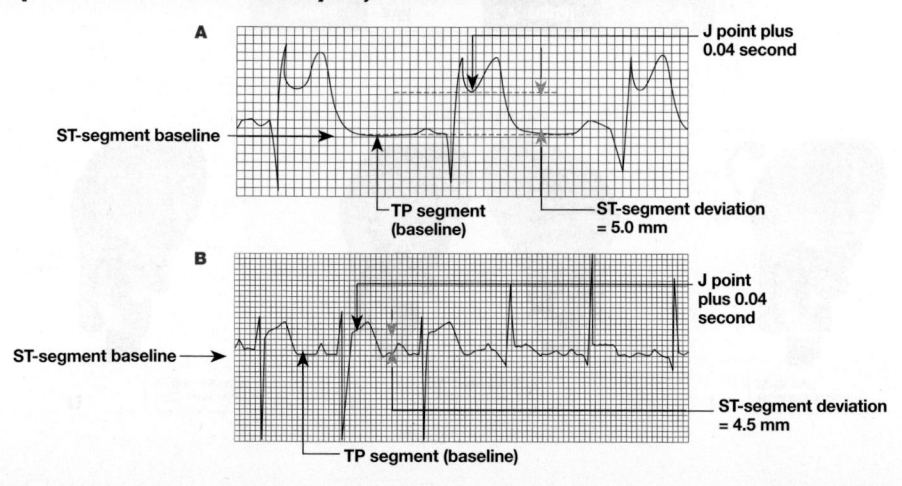

ECG Lead Changes Due to Injury or Infarct With Coronary Artery, Anatomic Area of Damage, and Associated Complications

Leads With ECG Changes	Injury/Infarct-Related Artery	Area of Damage	Associated Complications
V_1-V_2	LCA: LAD-septal branch	Septum, His bundle, bundle branches	Infranodal block and BBBs
V_3-V_4	LCA: LAD-diagonal branch	Anterior wall LV	LV dysfunction, CHF, BBBs, complete heart block, PVCs
V_5-V_6 plus I and aVL	LCA: circumflex branch	High lateral wall LV	LV dysfunction, AV nodal block in some
II, III, aVF	RCA: posterior descending branch	Inferior wall LV, posterior wall LV	Hypotension, sensitivity to nitroglycerin and morphine sulfate
V_4R (II, III, aVF)	RCA: proximal branches	RV, inferior wall LV, posterior wall LV	Hypotension, supranodal and AV-nodal blocks, atrial fibrillation/flutter, PACs, adverse medical reactions
V_1 through V_4 (marked depression)	Either LCA-circumflex or RCA-posterior descending branch	Posterior wall LV	LV dysfunction

LCA indicates left coronary artery; LAD, left anterior descending artery; RCA, right coronary artery; LV, left ventricle (left ventricular); RV, right ventricle; BBB, bundle branch block; CHF, congestive heart failure; PVC, premature ventricular complex; AV, atrioventricular; and PAC, premature atrial complex.

Acute ST-Segment Elevation
Potential Adjunctive Therapies (Do Not Delay Reperfusion to Administer)
β-Blockers

Rationale: Blocks sympathetic nervous system stimulation of heart rate and vasoconstriction. Decreases myocardial oxygen consumption and increases myocardial salvage in area of infarct and can reduce incidence of ventricular ectopy and fibrillation.

Caution: Early aggressive β-blockade poses a net hazard in hemodynamically unstable patients and should be avoided.

IV β-blockers should not be administered to STEMI or UA/NSTEMI patients who have *any* of the following:

1. **Signs of heart failure**
2. **Evidence of a low output state**
3. **Increased risk* for cardiogenic shock**
4. **Other relative contraindications to β-blockade (PR interval greater than 0.24 second, second- or third-degree heart block, active asthma, or reactive airway disease)**

*Risk factors for cardiogenic shock (the greater the number of risk factors present, the higher the risk of developing cardiogenic shock) are age >70 years, systolic blood pressure <120 mm Hg, sinus tachycardia >110/min or heart rate <60/min, and increased time since onset of symptoms of STEMI.

STEMI and UA/NSTEMI Recommendations

- Oral β-blocker therapy should be initiated in the first 24 hours for patients who do not have any of the 4 conditions listed above (Class I).
- It is reasonable to administer an *intravenous* β-blocker at the time of presentation to STEMI patients *who are hypertensive and who do not have any of the* 4 conditions listed above (Class IIa).
- Patients with early contraindications within the first 24 hours of STEMI should be reevaluated for candidacy for β-blocker therapy as secondary prevention. Patients with moderate or severe LV failure should receive β-blocker therapy as secondary prevention with a gradual titration scheme.

Heparin for Acute Coronary Syndromes

- *STEMI–Fibrinolytic Adjunct:* Anticoagulant therapy for a minimum of 48 hours and preferably the duration of hospitalization, up to 8 days. Regimens other than unfractionated heparin (UFH) are recommended if anticoagulant therapy is given for more than 48 hours. Recommended regimens include
  — UFH: Initial bolus 60 U/kg (maximum 4000 U) followed by intravenous infusion of 12 U/kg per hour (maximum 1000 U/hr) initially adjusted to maintain the aPTT at 50 to 70 seconds (duration of treatment 48 hours or until angiography).
  — Enoxaparin (provided serum creatinine <2.5 mg/dL in men and 2 mg/dL in women): If age <75 years, an initial bolus of 30 mg IV is followed 15 minutes later by SC injections 1 mg/kg every 12 hours. If age ≥75, the initial bolus is eliminated, and SC dose is reduced to 0.75 mg/kg every 12 hours. Regardless of age, if serum creatinine during course of treatment is estimated to be <30 mL/min (using Cockroft-Gault formula), the SC regimen is 1 mg/dL every 24 hours.
  — Fondaparinux (provided serum creatinine <3 mg/dL): Initial dose 2.5 mg IV; subsequent SC injections 2.5 mg ONCE daily. Maintenance dosing should be continued for duration of hospitalization, up to 8 days.
- *UA/NSTEMI:* For patients at high-to-intermediate risk, anticoagulant therapy should be added to antiplatelet therapy. Initial invasive strategy:
  — UFH: Loading dose 60 U/kg (maximum 4000 U) as bolus; maintenance infusion of 12 U/kg per hour to maintain aPTT 50 to 70 seconds.
  — Enoxaparin: Loading dose: 30 mg IV bolus. Maintenance dose: If creatinine clearance ≥30 mL/min, give 1 mg/kg SC every 12 hours. If creatinine clearance <30 mL/min, give 1 mg/kg once every 24 hours.
  — Fondaparinux: 2.5 mg/kg SC ONCE every 24 hours. Avoid if creatinine clearance <30 mL/min.
  — Bivalirudin: 0.1 mg/kg bolus; maintenance 0.25 mg/kg per hour infusion.

ST-Segment Elevation or New or Presumably New LBBB: Evaluation for Reperfusion

Step 1: Assess time and risk
- Time since onset of symptoms
- Risk of STEMI (TIMI Risk Score for STEMI)
- Risk of fibrinolysis
- Time required to transport to skilled PCI catheterization suite (first medical contact/door-to-balloon time)

Step 2: Select reperfusion (fibrinolysis or invasive) strategy
    Note: If presentation ≤3 hours from symptom onset and no delay for PCI, then no preference for either strategy.

Fibrinolysis is generally preferred if:	An invasive strategy is generally preferred if:
• Early presentation (≤3 hours from symptom onset and delay to PCI)	• Late presentation (symptom onset >3 hours ago)

• Invasive strategy is not an option (eg, lack of access to skilled PCI facility or difficult vascular access) or would be delayed
  — Medical contact–to-balloon or door-to-balloon >90 min
  — (Door-to-balloon) minus (door-to-needle) is >1 hour
	• Skilled PCI facility available with surgical backup
	  — Medical contact–to-balloon or door-to-balloon ≤90 min
	  — (Door-to-balloon) minus (door-to-needle) is ≤1 hour

• No contraindications to fibrinolysis	• Contraindications to fibrinolysis, including increased risk of bleeding and ICH
	• High risk from STEMI (CHF, Killip class is ≥3)
	• Diagnosis of STEMI is in doubt

Evaluate for Primary PCI (Percutaneous Coronary Intervention)

Can restore vessel patency and normal flow with >90% success in experienced high-volume centers with experienced providers

Primary PCI is most effective for the following:

- In cardiogenic shock patients (<75 years old) if performed ≤18 hours from onset of shock and ≤36 hours from onset of ST-elevation infarction. However, up to 40% of shock patients require CABG for optimal management.
- In selected patients >75 years old with STEMI and cardiogenic shock.
- In patients with indications for reperfusion but with a contraindication to fibrinolytic therapy.

Best results achieved at PCI centers with these characteristics:

- Centers with high volume (>200 PCI procedures/year; at least 36 are primary PCI).
- Experienced operator with technical skill.
- Balloon dilation ≤90 minutes from initial medical contact or ED presentation.
- Achievement of normal flow rate (TIMI-3) in >90% of cases without emergency CABG grafting, stroke, or death.
- At least 50% resolution of maximal ST-segment elevation (microvascular reperfusion).

Evaluate for Fibrinolytic Therapy: Assess Eligibility and Risk-Benefit Ratio

Early treatment (door-to-drug time ≤30 minutes) can limit infarct size, preserve LV function, reduce mortality.

- Maximum myocardial salvage occurs with early fibrinolytic administration, although a reduction in mortality may still be observed up to 12 hours from onset of continuous persistent symptoms.
- Normal flow achieved in 54% of patients treated with accelerated tPA, in 33% of patients treated with streptokinase and heparin.

Most effective in the following patients:

- Early presentation
- Larger infarction
- Younger patients with lower risk of intracerebral hemorrhage

Benefits with age and delayed presentation:

- Patients >75 years of age have increased risk of cerebral hemorrhage but absolute benefit similar to younger patients.
- Less benefit if presentation 12 to 24 hours or smaller infarction.

May be harmful:

- ST-segment depression (may be harmful and should not be used—unless true posterior MI present)
- Patients >24 hours after onset of pain
- Presence of high blood pressure (SBP >175 mm Hg) on presentation to the ED increases the risk of stroke after fibrinolytic therapy

Fibrinolytic Therapy
Contraindications for fibrinolytic use in STEMI consistent with ACC/AHA 2007 Focused Update*

Absolute Contraindications

- Any prior intracranial hemorrhage (ICH)
- Known structural cerebral vascular lesion (eg, AVM)
- Known malignant intracranial neoplasm (primary or metastatic)
- Ischemic stroke within 3 months EXCEPT acute ischemic stroke within 3 hours
- Suspected aortic dissection
- Active bleeding or bleeding diathesis (excluding menses)
- Significant closed head trauma or facial trauma within 3 months

Relative Contraindications

- History of chronic, severe, poorly controlled hypertension
- Severe uncontrolled hypertension on presentation (SBP >180 mm Hg or DBP >110 mm Hg)†
- History of prior ischemic stroke greater than 3 months, dementia, or known intracranial pathology not covered in contraindications
- Traumatic or prolonged (>10 minutes) CPR or major surgery (<3 weeks)
- Recent (within 2 to 4 weeks) internal bleeding
- Noncompressible vascular punctures
- For streptokinase/anistreplase: prior exposure (more than 5 days ago) or prior allergic reaction to these agents
- Pregnancy
- Active peptic ulcer
- Current use of anticoagulants: the higher the INR, the higher the risk of bleeding

SBP indicates systolic blood pressure; DBP, diastolic blood pressure; CPR, cardiopulmonary resuscitation; INR, International Normalized Ratio.

*Note: Viewed as advisory for clinical decision making and may not be all-inclusive or definitive.

†Could be an absolute contraindication in low-risk patients with myocardial infarction.

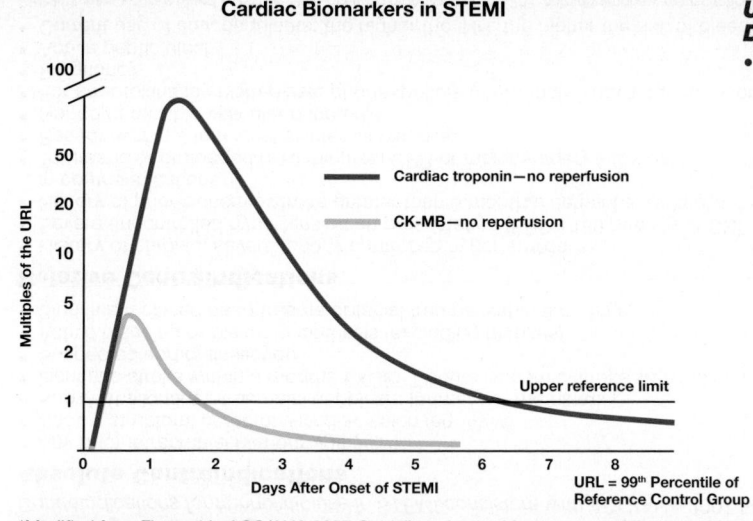

Cardiac Biomarkers in STEMI

Cardiac troponin—no reperfusion

CK-MB—no reperfusion

Upper reference limit

Multiples of the URL

Days After Onset of STEMI

URL = 99th Percentile of
Reference Control Group

Update: Universal Definition of AMI

- Detection of a rise and fall of cardiac biomarkers (preferably troponin) with at least one value above the 99th percentile of the upper reference limit (URL) and at least one of the following:
  - Symptoms of ischemia
  - ECG changes of ischemia: ST-T changes or new LBBB
  - Development of pathological Q waves
  - Imaging evidence of loss of viable myocardium or new regional wall motion abnormality

*Modified from Figure 4 in ACC/AHA 2007 Guidelines for the Management of Patients With Unstable Angina/Non–ST-Elevation Myocardial Infarction: Executive Summary. *Circulation*. 2007;116:827.

Cardiac Troponins

- Troponin I and troponin T cardiac-specific structural proteins not normally detected in serum. Patients with increased troponin levels have increased thrombus burden and microvascular embolization.
- Preferred biomarker for diagnosis of MI. Increased sensitivity compared with CK-MB. Elevation above 99th percentile of mean population value is diagnostic.
- Detect minimal myocardial damage in patients with UA/NSTEMI.
  - 30% of patients without ST-segment elevation who would otherwise be diagnosed with unstable angina have small amounts of myocardial damage when troponin assays are used (eg, CK-MB negative).
  - These patients are at increased risk for major adverse cardiac events and may benefit from new therapies such as GP IIb/IIIa inhibitors compared with patients who lack elevations in these cardiac-specific markers.
  - These patients are at increased risk for subsequent nonfatal MI and sudden cardiac death.
- Useful in risk stratification and prognosis: provides delayed confirmation of STEMI diagnosis in patients with ST-elevation; risk stratifies UA/NSTEMI.
- Biphasic release kinetics—elevated several days (replace LDH isoenzymes).

CK-MB

- Present in skeletal muscle and serum, less specific than troponin.
- Preferred marker for reinfarction and noninvasive assessment of reperfusion.

TIMI Risk Score for Patients With Unstable Angina and Non–ST-Segment Elevation MI: Predictor Variables

Predictor Variable	Point Value of Variable	Definition
Age ≥65	1	
≥3 risk factors for CAD	1	**Risk factors:** • Family history of CAD • Hypertension • Hypercholesterolemia • Diabetes • Current smoker
Aspirin use in last 7 days	1	
Recent, severe symptoms of angina	1	≥2 anginal events in last 24 hours
Elevated cardiac markers	1	CK-MB or cardiac-specific troponin level

ST deviation ≥0.5 mm	1	ST depression ≥0.5 mm is significant; transient ST elevation ≥0.5 mm for <20 minutes is treated as ST-segment depression and is high risk; ST elevation >1 mm for more than 20 minutes places these patients in the STEMI treatment category.
Prior coronary artery stenosis ≥50%	1	Risk predictor remains valid even if this information is unknown

Calculated TIMI Risk Score	Risk of ≥1 Primary End Point* in ≤14 Days	Risk Status
0 or 1	5%	Low
2	8%	Low
3	13%	Intermediate
4	20%	Intermediate
5	26%	High
6 or 7	41%	High

*Primary end points: death, new or recurrent MI, or need for urgent revascularization.

Risk Stratification and Treatment Strategies for Patients With UA/NSTEMI

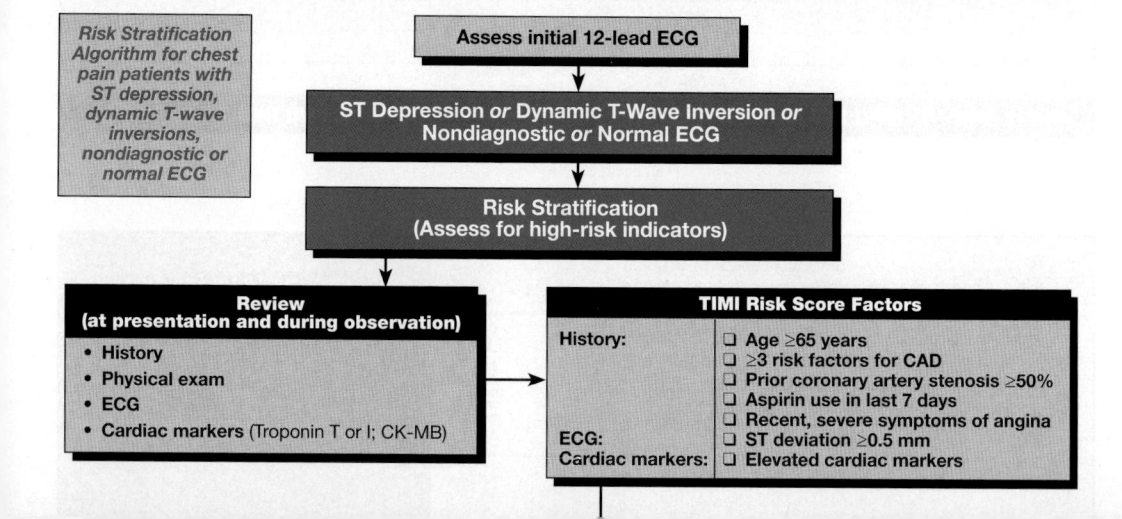

Risk Stratification Algorithm for chest pain patients with ST depression, dynamic T-wave inversions, nondiagnostic or normal ECG

Assess initial 12-lead ECG

ST Depression *or* Dynamic T-Wave Inversion *or* Nondiagnostic *or* Normal ECG

Risk Stratification
(Assess for high-risk indicators)

Review
(at presentation and during observation)
- History
- Physical exam
- ECG
- Cardiac markers (Troponin T or I; CK-MB)

TIMI Risk Score Factors

History:	☐ Age ≥65 years
	☐ ≥3 risk factors for CAD
	☐ Prior coronary artery stenosis ≥50%
	☐ Aspirin use in last 7 days
	☐ Recent, severe symptoms of angina
ECG:	☐ ST deviation ≥0.5 mm
Cardiac markers:	☐ Elevated cardiac markers

Review for ACC/AHA High-Risk Indicators (in addition to the TIMI risk factors)	
History:	❏ High (≥5) or Intermediate (3 or 4) TIMI risk score* ❏ PCI or prior CABG within 6 months
Physical Exam:	❏ Recurrent angina/ischemia with CHF symptoms, an S_3 gallop, pulmonary edema, worsening rales, or new or worsening mitral regurgitation
ECG and Cardiac Markers:	❏ Hemodynamic or electrical instability (ischemic VT) ❏ Elevated cardiac markers
Evaluation:	❏ High-risk findings on noninvasive stress testing ❏ Depressed LV systolic function (eg, EF <0.40 on noninvasive study)
*Note TIMI risk score should be derived by experienced physicians. Application to all patients with chest discomfort is not indicated.	

Does patient stratify as *high* or *intermediate risk* by one or more of the following:

❏ ST deviation? (original or subsequent ECG)
❏ TIMI Risk Score ≥5?
❏ TIMI Risk Score 3 or 4?
❏ Cardiac markers elevated?
❏ Age ≥75?
❏ Unstable angina (UA)?
❏ ACC/AHA high-risk indicator?

High-Intermediate Risk: Invasive Strategy ← YES ———————————— NO → **Low Risk: Conservative Strategy†**

†No benefit for early invasive strategy in low-risk women (may be excess risk with invasive strategy).

Treatment Recommendations for UA/NSTEMI

Glycoprotein IIb/IIIa Inhibitors

Recommendations

Expert consultation advised

Actions

- Inhibits the *integrin GP IIb/IIIa receptor* in the membrane of platelets.
- Inhibits final common pathway activation of platelet aggregation.

Clinical trials

- Major benefit occurs in patients who are troponin positive in whom invasive strategy selected.

Available approved agents

- *Abciximab* (ReoPro): a murine monoclonal antibody to the GP IIb/IIIa receptor.
  - FDA-approved for patients with UA/NSTEMI or unstable angina and *planned* PCI within 24 hours.
- *Eptifibatide* (Integrilin): small-molecule cyclical heptapeptide that binds to the receptor; short half-life.
- *Tirofiban* (Aggrastat): small-molecule nonpeptide, also with short half-life.
  - Efficacy demonstrated in randomized clinical trial with early use and PCI strategy.

Clopidogrel

Recommendations

STEMI (Class I)

- Clopidogrel 75 mg per day orally should be added to aspirin for patients receiving fibrinolytic therapy and those who do not receive reperfusion therapy. Treatment should be continued for at least 14 days.
- In patients for whom CABG is planned, the drug should be withheld for at least 5 days and preferably for 7 days unless the urgency for revascularization outweighs the risk of excess bleeding.

STEMI (Class II)

- In patients <75 years of age, it is reasonable to administer a loading dose of 300 mg.
- Long-term maintenance therapy (eg, 1 year with clopidogrel 75 mg daily) is reasonable.

UA/NSTEMI (Class I)

- For UA/NSTEMI patients treated medically, clopidogrel (75 mg/day orally) should be prescribed for at least 1 month and ideally for up to 1 year.
- Clopidogrel is indicated for patients allergic to aspirin.

Following PCI with STENT

- Use current stent-specific prophylaxis, eg, bare metal stent (BMS), drug eluting stent (DES).

Conveying News of a Sudden Death to Family Members

- Call the family if they have not been notified. Explain that their loved one has been admitted to the ED or critical care unit and that the situation is serious. If possible, survivors should be told of the death in person, not over the telephone.
- Obtain as much information as possible about the patient and the circumstances surrounding the death. Carefully go over the events as they happened in the ED.
- When family arrives, ask someone to take family members to a private area. Walk in, introduce yourself, and sit down. Address the closest relative.
- Briefly describe the circumstances leading to the death. Go over the sequence of events in the ED. Avoid euphemisms such as "he's passed on," "she's no longer with us," or "he's left us." Instead use the words "death," "dying," or "dead."
- Allow time for the shock to be absorbed. Make eye contact, touch, and share. Convey your feelings with a phrase such as "You have my (our) sincere sympathy" rather than "I am (we are) sorry."

- Determine the patient's suitability for and wishes about organ or tissue donation (use driver's license and patient records). Discuss with family if possible.
- Allow as much time as necessary for questions and discussion. Go over the events several times to make sure everything is understood and to facilitate further questions.
- Allow the family the opportunity to see their relative. If equipment is still connected, let the family know.
- Know in advance what happens next and who will sign the death certificate. Physicians may impose burdens on staff and family if they fail to understand policies about death certification and disposition of the body. Know the answers to these questions before meeting the family.
- Enlist the aid of a social worker or the clergy if not already present.
- Offer to contact the patient's attending or family physician and to be available if there are further questions. Arrange for follow-up and continued support during the grieving period.

Family Presence During Resuscitation

According to surveys in the United States and the United Kingdom, most family members would like to be present during the attempted resuscitation of a loved one. Parents and care providers of chronically ill patients are often knowledgeable about and comfortable with medical equipment and emergency procedures. Even family members with no medical background report that being at the side of a loved one and saying goodbye during the final moments of life is extremely comforting. Family members often do not ask if they can be present, but healthcare providers should offer the opportunity whenever possible.

When family members are present during resuscitative efforts, resuscitation team members should be sensitive to the presence of the family. If possible, one team member should remain with the family to answer questions, clarify information, and comfort the family.

Administration Notes

Peripheral IV:	Resuscitation drugs administered via peripheral IV catheter should be followed by bolus of 20 mL IV fluid to move drug into central circulation. Then elevate extremity for 10 to 20 seconds.
Intraosseous:	ACLS drugs that can be administered by IV route can be administered by intraosseous (IO) route.
Endotracheal:	Drugs that can be administered by endotracheal route are indicated. Optimal endotracheal doses have not yet been established. IV/IO administration is preferred because it provides more reliable drug delivery and pharmacologic effect. Medication delivered via endotracheal tube should be diluted in water or NS to a volume of 5 to 10 mL. Provide several positive-pressure breaths after medication is instilled.

Drug/Therapy	Indications/Precautions	Adult Dosage
ACE Inhibitors (Angiotensin-Converting Enzyme Inhibitors)	**Indications** • ACE inhibitors reduce mortality and improve LV dysfunction in post-AMI patients. They help prevent adverse LV remodeling, delay progression of heart failure, and decrease sudden death and recurrent MI. • An ACE inhibitor should be administered orally within the first 24 hours after onset of symptoms and continued long term. • Clinical heart failure without hypotension in patients not responding to digitalis or diuretics. • Clinical signs of AMI with LV dysfunction. • LV ejection fraction <40%.	**Approach**: ACE inhibitor therapy should start with low-dose oral administration (with possible IV doses for some preparations) and increase steadily to achieve a full dose within 24 to 48 hours. An angiotensin receptor blocker (ARB) should be administered to patients intolerant of ACE inhibitors.
(continued)		

Enalapril	**Precautions/Contraindications for All ACE Inhibitors**	**Enalapril (IV = Enalaprilat)**

Enalapril

Precautions/Contraindications for All ACE Inhibitors

- *Contraindicated* in pregnancy (may cause fetal injury or death).
- Contraindicated in angioedema.
- Hypersensitivity to ACE inhibitors.
- Reduce dose in renal failure (creatinine >2.5 mg/dL in men, >2 mg/dL in women). Avoid in bilateral renal artery stenosis.
- Serum potassium >5 mEq/L

Captopril

- Do not give if patient is hypotensive (SBP <100 mm Hg or more than 30 mm Hg below baseline) or volume depleted.

Lisinopril

- Generally not started in ED; after reperfusion therapy has been completed and blood pressure has stabilized, start within 24 hours.

Ramipril

Enalapril (IV = Enalaprilat)
- PO: Start with a single dose of 2.5 mg. Titrate to 20 mg PO BID.
- IV: 1.25 mg IV initial dose over 5 minutes, then 1.25 to 5 mg IV every 6 hours.
- IV form is contraindicated in STEMI (risk of hypotension).

Captopril, AMI Dose
- Start with a single dose of 6.25 mg PO.
- Advance to 25 mg TID and then to 50 mg TID as tolerated.

Lisinopril, AMI Dose
- 5 mg within 24 hours of onset of symptoms, then
- 5 mg given after 24 hours, then
- 10 mg given after 48 hours, then
- 10 mg once daily

Ramipril
- Start with a single dose of 2.5 mg PO. Titrate to 5 mg PO BID as tolerated.

Drug/Therapy	Indications/Precautions	Adult Dosage
Adenosine	**Indications** • First drug for most forms of stable narrow-complex SVT. Effective in terminating those due to reentry involving AV node or sinus node. • May consider for unstable narrow-complex reentry tachycardia while preparations made for cardioversion. • Wide-complex regular tachycardia, thought to be or previously defined to be, reentry SVT. • Does *not* convert atrial fibrillation, atrial flutter, or VT. • Diagnostic maneuver: stable narrow-complex SVT. **Precautions/Contraindications** • Contraindicated in poison/drug-induced tachycardia or second- or third-degree heart block. • Transient side effects include flushing, chest pain or tightness, brief periods of asystole or bradycardia, ventricular ectopy. • Less effective (larger doses may be required) in patients taking theophylline or caffeine. • Reduce dose to 3 mg in patients receiving dipyridamole or carbamazepine. • If administered for wide-complex tachycardia/VT, may cause deterioration (including hypotension). • Transient periods of sinus bradycardia and ventricular ectopy are common after termination of SVT. • Safe and effective in pregnancy.	**IV Rapid Push** • Place patient in mild reverse Trendelenburg position before administration of drug. • Initial bolus of 6 mg given *rapidly* over 1 to 3 seconds followed by NS bolus of 20 mL; then elevate the extremity. • A second dose (12 mg) can be given in 1 to 2 minutes if needed. • A third dose (12 mg) may be given in 1 to 2 minutes if needed. **Injection Technique** • Record rhythm strip during administration. • Draw up adenosine dose and flush in 2 separate syringes. • Attach both syringes to the IV injection port closer to patient. • Clamp IV tubing above injection port. • Push IV adenosine *as quickly as possible* (1 to 3 seconds). • While maintaining pressure on adenosine plunger, push NS flush *as rapidly as possible* after adenosine. • Unclamp IV tubing.

Amiodarone

Amiodarone is a complex drug with effects on sodium, potassium, and calcium channels as well as α-and β-adrenergic blocking properties. Patients must be hospitalized while the loading doses of amiodarone are administered. Amiodarone should be prescribed only by physicians who are experienced in the treatment of life-threatening arrhythmias, thoroughly familiar with amiodarone's risks and benefits, and have access to laboratory facilities capable of adequately monitoring the effectiveness and side effects of amiodarone treatment.

Indications

Because its use is associated with toxicity, amiodarone is indicated for use in patients with life-threatening arrhythmias when administered with appropriate monitoring:

- VF/pulseless VT unresponsive to shock delivery, CPR, and a vasopressor
- Recurrent, hemodynamically unstable VT

With expert consultation amiodarone may be used for treatment of some atrial and ventricular arrhythmias.

Other Uses: Seek Expert Consultation
Caution: Multiple complex drug interactions

VF/VT Cardiac Arrest Unresponsive to CPR, Shock, and Vasopressor

300 mg IV/IO push (recommend dilution in 20 to 30 mL D$_5$W). Initial dose can be followed by ONE 150 mg IV push in 3 to 5 minutes.

Life-Threatening Arrhythmias

Maximum cumulative dose: 2.2 g IV/24 h.
May be administered as follows:
- *Rapid infusion:* 150 mg IV over first 10 minutes (15 mg/min). May repeat rapid infusion (150 mg IV) every 10 minutes as needed.
- *Slow infusion:* 360 mg IV over 6 hours (1 mg/min).
- *Maintenance infusion:* 540 mg IV over 18 hours (0.5 mg/min).

Precautions

- With multiple dosing, cumulative doses >2.2 g/24 hours are associated with significant hypotension in clinical trials.
- Do not administer with other drugs that prolong QT interval (eg, procainamide).
- Terminal elimination is extremely long (half-life lasts up to 40 days).

Advanced Cardiovascular Life Support Drugs and Electrical Therapy

Drug/Therapy	Indications/Precautions	Adult Dosage
Amrinone *(See Inamrinone)*		
Aspirin	**Indications** • Administer to all patients with ACS, particularly reperfusion candidates, unless hypersensitive to aspirin. • Blocks formation of thromboxane A_2, which causes platelets to aggregate and arteries to constrict. This reduces overall ACS mortality, reinfarction, nonfatal stroke. • Any person with symptoms ("pressure," "heavy weight," "squeezing," "crushing") suggestive of ischemic pain. **Precautions** • Relatively contraindicated in patients with active ulcer disease or asthma. • Contraindicated in patients with known hypersensitivity to aspirin.	• 160 mg to 325 mg nonenteric coated tablet as soon as possible (chewing is preferable). • May use rectal suppository (300 mg) for patients who cannot take PO.

Atropine Sulfate

Can be given via endotracheal tube

Administration should not delay pacing for severely symptomatic patients

Indications
- First drug for symptomatic sinus bradycardia.
- May be beneficial in presence of AV nodal block or ventricular asystole. **Will not be effective for infranodal (Mobitz type II) block.**
- Second drug (after epinephrine or vasopressin) for asystole or bradycardic pulseless electrical activity.
- Organophosphate (eg, nerve agent) poisoning: extremely large doses may be needed.

Precautions
- Use with caution in presence of myocardial ischemia and hypoxia. Increases myocardial oxygen demand.
- Avoid in hypothermic bradycardia.
- Will not be effective for infranodal (type II) AV block and new third-degree block with wide QRS complexes. (In these patients may cause paradoxical slowing. Be prepared to pace or give catecholamines.)
- Doses of atropine <0.5 mg may result in paradoxical slowing of heart rate.

Asystole or Pulseless Electrical Activity
- 1 mg IV/IO push.
- May repeat every 3 to 5 minutes (if asystole persists) to a maximum of 3 doses (3 mg).

Bradycardia (with or without ACS)
- 0.5 mg IV every 3 to 5 minutes as needed, not to exceed total dose of 0.04 mg/kg (total 3 mg).
- Use shorter dosing interval (3 minutes) and higher doses in severe clinical conditions.

Endotracheal Administration
- 2 to 3 mg diluted in 10 mL water or NS.

Organophosphate Poisoning
Extremely large doses (2 to 4 mg or higher) may be needed.

Drug/Therapy	Indications/Precautions	Adult Dosage
β-Blockers **Metoprolol tartrate** **Atenolol** **Propranolol**	**Indications (Apply to all β-blockers)** • Administer to all patients with suspected myocardial infarction and unstable angina in the absence of contraindication. These are effective antianginal agents and can reduce incidence of VF. • Useful as an adjunctive agent with fibrinolytic therapy. May reduce nonfatal reinfarction and recurrent ischemia. • To convert to normal sinus rhythm or to slow ventricular response (or both) in supraventricular tachyarrhythmias (re-entry SVT, atrial fibrillation, or atrial flutter). β-blockers are second-line agents after adenosine. • To reduce myocardial ischemia and damage in AMI patients with elevated heart rate, blood pressure, or both. • For emergency antihypertensive therapy for hemorrhagic and acute ischemic stroke. **Precautions/Contraindications (Apply to all β-blockers unless noted)** • Early aggressive beta blockade may be hazardous in hemodynamically unstable patients.	**Metoprolol tartrate (AMI regimen)** • Initial IV dose: 5 mg slow IV at 5-minute intervals to a total of 15 mg. • Oral regimen to follow IV dose: 50 mg BID for 24 hours, then increase to 100 mg BID. **Atenolol (AMI regimen)** • 5 mg slow IV (over 5 minutes). • Wait 10 minutes, then give second dose of 5 mg slow IV (over 5 minutes). • In 10 minutes, if tolerated well, may start 50 mg PO; then give 50 mg PO q 12 h × 2, then 100 mg daily. **Propranolol** • Total dose: 0.1 mg/kg by slow IV push, divided into 3 equal doses at 2- to 3-minute intervals. Do not exceed 1 mg/min. • Repeat in 2 minutes after total dose is given if necessary.

(continued) ↓

Esmolol

- Do not give to patients with STEMI if any of the following is present:
  - Signs of heart failure
  - Low cardiac output
  - Increased risk for cardiogenic shock
- Relative contraindications include PR interval >0.24 second, second- or third-degree heart block, active asthma, reactive airway disease, severe bradycardia, systolic BP <100 mm Hg.
- Concurrent IV administration with IV calcium channel blocking agents like verapamil or diltiazem can cause severe hypotension.
- Monitor cardiac and pulmonary status during administration.
- Propranolol is contraindicated in cocaine-induced ACS.

Labetalol

Esmolol
- 0.5 mg/kg over 1 minute, followed by 4-minute infusion at 50 µg/kg (0.05 mg/kg) per minute; maximum: 0.3 mg/kg per minute for a total of 200 µg/kg.
- If initial response is inadequate, give second 0.5 mg/kg bolus over 1 minute, then increase infusion to 100 µg/kg per minute; max infusion rate 300 µg/kg (0.3 mg/kg) per minute.
- Esmolol has a short half-life (2 to 9 minutes).

Labetalol
- 10 mg labetalol IV push over 1 to 2 minutes.
- May repeat or double labetalol every 10 minutes to a maximum dose of 150 mg, or give initial dose as a bolus, then start labetalol infusion at 2 to 8 mg/min.

Calcium Chloride

10% solution is 100 mg/mL in 10 mL

Indications
- Known or suspected hyperkalemia (eg, renal failure).
- Ionized hypocalcemia (eg, after multiple blood transfusions).
- As an antidote for toxic effects (hypotension and arrhythmias) from calcium channel blocker overdose or β-blocker overdose.

Precautions
- Do not use routinely in cardiac arrest.
- Do not mix with sodium bicarbonate.

Typical Dose
- 500 mg to 1000 mg (5 to 10 mL of a 10% solution) IV for hyperkalemia and calcium channel blocker overdose. May be repeated as needed.

Drug/Therapy	Indications/Precautions	Adult Dosage
Cardioversion (Synchronized) Administered via adhesive defibrillation electrodes or handheld paddles from a defibrillator/monitor Place defibrillator/monitor in synchronized (sync) mode Sync mode delivers energy just after the R wave	**Indications** • All tachycardias (rate >150 per minute) with serious signs and symptoms related to the tachycardia. • May give brief trial of medications based on specific arrhythmias. **Precautions/Contraindications** • **Contraindications:** Poison/drug-induced tachycardia. • In critical conditions go to immediate unsynchronized shocks. • Urgent cardioversion is generally not needed if heart rate is ≤150 per minute. • Reactivation of sync mode is required after each attempted cardioversion (defibrillators/cardioverters default to unsynchronized mode). • Prepare to defibrillate immediately if cardioversion causes VF. • Synchronized cardioversion cannot be performed unless the patient is connected to monitor leads; lead select switch must be on lead I, II, or III and not on "paddles."	**Technique** • Premedicate whenever possible. • Engage sync mode before each attempt. • Look for sync markers on the R wave. • Clear the patient before each shock. • Reentry SVT and atrial flutter often respond to lower energy levels; start with 50 J to 100 J. If initial dose fails, increase in stepwise fashion. • For atrial fibrillation, use 100 to 200 J initial monophasic shock, or 100 to 120 J initial (selected) biphasic shock, and then increase in stepwise fashion. • Deliver monophasic shocks in the following sequence: 100 J, 200 J, 300 J, 360 J. Use this sequence for monomorphic VT. • Treat unstable polymorphic VT (irregular form and rate) with high-energy *unsynchronized* dose used for VF: 360 J monophasic waveform or biphasic device-specific defibrillation dose. ↓

(continued)

- Press "charge" button, "clear" the patient, and press both "shock" buttons simultaneously. Be prepared to perform CPR or defibrillation.

Clopidogrel

Indications

Used for antiplatelet therapy; especially useful for patients who cannot tolerate ASA.

- STEMI: Add to aspirin for all patients receiving fibrinolytic therapy and those not receiving reperfusion therapy; continue at least 14 days.
- Following PCI with stent: Use stent-specific prophylaxis.

Precautions

- Do not administer to patients with active pathologic bleeding (eg, peptic ulcer). Use with caution in patients with risk of bleeding.
- Use with caution in the presence of hepatic impairment.
- **When CABG is planned, withhold drug for 5 to 7 days unless need for revascularization is urgent.**

Dose

- STEMI patient <75 years: administer loading dose of 300 mg PO, followed by maintenance dose of 75 mg PO q day for at least 1 month and ideally up to 1 year; full effects will not develop for several days.
- UA/NSTEMI: 75 mg PO daily for 1 month, ideally up to 1 year.

Drug/Therapy	Indications/Precautions	Adult Dosage
Defibrillation **Single Shock Sequence, Resume CPR Immediately** Use conventional monitor/defibrillator (ACLS provider) Use automated or shock advisory defibrillator (AED)—lay rescuer and BLS healthcare provider Administer shocks via remote adhesive electrodes or handheld paddles	**Indications** First intervention for VF or pulseless VT. **Precautions** • Always "clear" the patient before discharging a defibrillation shock. • Do not delay defibrillation for VF/VT if witnessed arrest and defibrillator is available. • EMS providers who do not witness arrest may provide 5 cycles (about 2 minutes) of CPR before attempting defibrillation. • Do not shock asystole. • Treat VF/VT in hypothermic cardiac arrest with an initial defibrillation shock. Repeat shocks for VF/VT only after core temperature rises above 30°C. • If patient in VF/VT has an automatic implantable cardioverter defibrillator (ICD), and ICD is delivering shocks, wait 30 to 60 seconds for completion of cycle.	**Adult Monophasic Defibrillation Energy Levels** • 360 J for first and subsequent monophasic shocks. **Manual Biphasic Defibrillator** • Use device-specific dose, typically selected energy of 120 J (rectilinear) or 150 J (truncated) to 200 J. • If unknown, use 200 J. Subsequent shocks: same or higher energy. **Following Single Shock** • Resume CPR, beginning with chest compressions, for 5 cycles or about 2 minutes, then reanalyze rhythm, deliver shock if needed, resume CPR. • If first 2 shocks fail to convert VF/VT, administer epinephrine or vasopressin. • If these medications fail to convert VF/VT, consider antiarrhythmic medications. *Note:* When using AED pads, do not use child pads or child attenuator system for adult defibrillation.

(continued)

↓   ↓

Defibrillation *(continued)*	• If patient has implanted device (eg pacer, ICD), place paddles and pads at least 1 inch (2.5 cm) from the device.	*Note:* Use adult pads and dose when child is 8 years of age and older, over 25 kg (55 pounds), or over 50 inches in length.

Digibind (Digoxin-Specific Antibody Therapy) 40 mg vial (each vial binds about 0.6 mg digoxin)	**Indications** Digoxin toxicity with the following: • Life-threatening arrhythmias. • Shock or congestive heart failure. • Hyperkalemia (potassium level >5 mEq/L). • Steady-state serum levels >10 to 15 ng/mL for symptomatic patients. **Precautions** • Serum digoxin levels rise after digibind therapy and should not be used to guide continuing therapy.	**Chronic Intoxication** 3 to 5 vials may be effective. **Acute Overdose** • IV dose varies according to amount of digoxin ingested. • Average dose is 10 vials (400 mg); may require up to 20 vials (800 mg). • See package insert for details.

Digoxin 0.25 mg/mL or 0.1 mg/mL supplied in 1 or 2 mL ampule (totals = 0.1 to 0.5 mg)	**Indications (may be of limited use)** • To slow ventricular response in atrial fibrillation or atrial flutter. • Alternative drug for reentry SVT. **Precautions** • Toxic effects are common and are frequently associated with serious arrhythmias. • Avoid electrical cardioversion if patient is receiving digoxin unless condition is life-threatening; use lower dose (10 to 20 J).	**IV Administration** • Loading doses of 10 to 15 µg/kg lean body weight provide therapeutic effect with minimum risk of toxic effects. • Repeat digoxin levels no sooner than 4 hours with IV dose; no sooner than 6 hours after oral dose. • Maintenance dose is affected by body mass and renal function. • Caution: Amiodarone interaction. Reduce digoxin dose by 50% when initiating amiodarone.

Advanced Cardiovascular Life Support Drugs and Electrical Therapy

Drug/Therapy	Indications/Precautions	Adult Dosage
Diltiazem	**Indications** • To control ventricular rate in atrial fibrillation and atrial flutter. May terminate reentrant arrhythmias that require AV nodal conduction for their continuation. • Use after adenosine to treat refractory reentry SVT in patients with narrow QRS complex and adequate blood pressure. **Precautions** • Do not use calcium channel blockers for wide-QRS tachycardias of uncertain origin or for poison/drug-induced tachycardia. • Avoid calcium channel blockers in patients with Wolff-Parkinson-White syndrome plus rapid atrial fibrillation or flutter, in patients with sick sinus syndrome, or in patients with AV block without a pacemaker. • Caution: Blood pressure may drop from peripheral vasodilation (greater drop with verapamil than with diltiazem).	**Acute Rate Control** • 15 to 20 mg (0.25 mg/kg) IV over 2 minutes. • May give another IV dose in 15 minutes at 20 to 25 mg (0.35 mg/kg) over 2 minutes. **Maintenance Infusion** 5 to 15 mg/h, titrated to physiologically appropriate heart rate (can dilute in D_5W or NS).

(continued)

Diltiazem *(continued)*	• Avoid in patients receiving oral β-blockers. • Concurrent IV administration with IV β-blockers can cause severe hypotension.	
Dobutamine *IV infusion*	**Indications** • Consider for pump problems (congestive heart failure, pulmonary congestion) with systolic blood pressure of 70 to 100 mm Hg and *no* signs of shock. **Precautions/Contraindications** • **Contraindication:** Suspected or known poison/drug-induced shock. • Avoid with systolic blood pressure <100 mm Hg and signs of shock. • May cause tachyarrhythmias, fluctuations in blood pressure, headache, and nausea. • Do not mix with sodium bicarbonate.	**IV Administration** • Usual infusion rate is 2 to 20 µg/kg per minute. • Titrate so heart rate does not increase by >10% of baseline. • Hemodynamic monitoring is recommended for optimal use. • Elderly patients may have a significantly decreased response.

Drug/Therapy	Indications/Precautions	Adult Dosage
Dopamine *IV infusion*	**Indications** • Second-line drug for symptomatic bradycardia (after atropine). • Use for hypotension (systolic blood pressure ≤70 to 100 mm Hg) with signs and symptoms of shock. **Precautions** • Correct hypovolemia with volume replacement before initiating dopamine. • Use with caution in cardiogenic shock with accompanying CHF. • May cause tachyarrhythmias, excessive vasoconstriction. • Do not mix with sodium bicarbonate.	**IV Administration** • Usual infusion rate is 2 to 20 µg/kg per minute. • Titrate to patient response, taper slowly.

Epinephrine

Can be given via endotracheal tube

Note: Available in 1:10 000 and 1:1000 concentrations

Indications
- **Cardiac arrest:** VF, pulseless VT, asystole, pulseless electrical activity.
- **Symptomatic bradycardia:** Can be considered after atropine as an alternative infusion to dopamine.
- **Severe hypotension:** Can be used when pacing and atropine fail, when hypotension accompanies bradycardia, or with phosphodiesterase enzyme inhibitor.
- **Anaphylaxis, severe allergic reactions:** Combine with large fluid volume, corticosteroids, antihistamines.

Precautions
- Raising blood pressure and increasing heart rate may cause myocardial ischemia, angina, and increased myocardial oxygen demand.
- High doses do not improve survival or neurologic outcome and may contribute to postresuscitation myocardial dysfunction.
- Higher doses *may* be required to treat poison/drug-induced shock.

Cardiac Arrest
- **IV/IO Dose:** 1 mg (10 mL of 1:10 000 solution) administered every 3 to 5 minutes during resuscitation. Follow each dose with 20 mL flush, elevate arm for 10 to 20 seconds after dose.
- **Higher Dose:** Higher doses (up to 0.2 mg/kg) may be used for specific indications (β-blocker or calcium channel blocker overdose)
- **Continuous Infusion:** Add 1 mg epinephrine (1 mL of 1:1000 solution) to 500 mL NS or D_5W. Initial infusion rate of 1 µg/min titrated to effect (typical dose: 2 to 10 µg/min).
- **Endotracheal Route** 2 to 2.5 mg diluted in 10 mL NS.

Profound Bradycardia or Hypotension
2 to 10 µg/min infusion; titrate to patient response.

Drug/Therapy	Indications/Precautions	Adult Dosage

Fibrinolytic Agents
 	
Alteplase, recombinant (Activase); tissue plasminogen activator (tPA)
 	
50 and 100 mg vials reconstituted with sterile water to 1 mg/mL
 	
For all 4 agents, use 2 peripheral IV lines, 1 line exclusively for fibrinolytic administration
 	
(continued)
	Indications
	For Cardiac Arrest: Insufficent evidence to recommend routine use.
	For AMI in Adults (see ACS section):
	• ST elevation (>1 mm in ≥2 contiguous leads) or new or presumably new LBBB.
	• In context of signs and symptoms of AMI.
	• Time from onset of symptoms ≤12 hours.
	For Acute Ischemic Stroke:
	(Alteplase is the only fibrinolytic agent approved for acute ischemic stroke. See Stroke section.)
	• Sudden onset of focal neurologic deficits or alterations in consciousness (eg, facial droop, arm drift, abnormal speech).
	• Absence of intracerebral or subarachnoid hemorrhage or mass effect on CT scan.
	• Absence of variable or rapidly improving neurologic deficits.
	• Alteplase can be started in <3 hours from symptom onset.
	↓
		Alteplase, recombinant (tPA)
		Recommended total dose is based on patient's weight.
		
		For STEMI:
		• Accelerated infusion (1.5 hours)
		  — Give 15 mg IV bolus.
		  — Then 0.75 mg/kg over next 30 minutes (not to exceed 50 mg).
		  — Then 0.5 mg/kg over 60 minutes (not to exceed 35 mg).
		  — Maximum total dose: 100 mg
		
		For Acute Ischemic Stroke:
		• Give 0.9 mg/kg (maximum 90 mg) infused over 60 minutes.
		• Give 10% of the total dose as an initial IV bolus over 1 minute.
		• Give the remaining 90% over the next 60 minutes.

Reteplase, recombinant (Retavase)
10 U vials reconstituted with sterile water to 1 U/mL

Streptokinase (Streptase)
Reconstitute to 1 mg/mL

Tenecteplase (TNKase)

Precautions and Exclusion Criteria
- Active internal bleeding (except menses) within 21 days.
- History of cerebrovascular, intracranial, or intraspinal event within 3 months (stroke, arteriovenous malformation, neoplasm, aneurysm, recent trauma, recent surgery).
- Major surgery or serious trauma within 14 days.
- Aortic dissection.
- Severe, uncontrolled hypertension.
- Known bleeding disorders.
- Prolonged CPR with evidence of thoracic trauma.
- Lumbar puncture within 7 days.
- Recent arterial puncture at noncompressible site.
- During the first 24 hours of fibrinolytic therapy for ischemic stroke, do not administer aspirin or heparin.

Reteplase, recombinant
- Give first 10 U IV bolus over 2 minutes.
- 30 minutes later give second 10 U IV bolus over 2 minutes. (Give NS flush before and after each bolus.)
- Give heparin and aspirin conjunctively.

Streptokinase
1.5 million U in a 1-hour infusion.

Tenecteplase
Bolus: 30 to 50 mg, weight adjusted.

Drug/Therapy	Indications/Precautions	Adult Dosage
Flumazenil	**Indications** Reverse respiratory depression and sedative effects from pure benzodiazepine overdose. **Precautions** • Effects may not outlast effect of benzodiazepines. • Monitor for recurrent respiratory depression. • Do not use in suspected tricyclic overdose. • Do not use in seizure-prone patients. • Do not use in unknown drug overdose or mixed drug overdose with drugs known to cause seizures (tricyclic antidepressants, cocaine, amphetamines, etc).	**First Dose** 0.2 mg IV over 15 seconds. **Second Dose** 0.3 mg IV over 30 seconds. If no adequate response, give third dose. **Third Dose** 0.5 mg IV given over 30 seconds. If no adequate response, repeat once every minute until adequate response or a total of 3 mg is given.

Furosemide

Indications
- For adjuvant therapy of acute pulmonary edema in patients with systolic blood pressure >90 to 100 mm Hg (without signs and symptoms of shock).
- Hypertensive emergencies.
- Increased intracranial pressure.

Precautions
Dehydration, hypovolemia, hypotension, hypokalemia, or other electrolyte imbalance may occur.

IV Administration
- 0.5 to 1 mg/kg given over 1 to 2 minutes.
- If no response, double dose to 2 mg/kg, slowly over 1 to 2 minutes.
- For new onset pulmonary edema with hypovolemia: <0.5 mg/kg.

Glucagon
Powdered in 1 and 10 mg vials

Reconstitute with provided solution

Indications
Adjuvant treatment of toxic effects of calcium channel blocker or β-blocker.

Precautions
- Do not mix with saline.
- May cause vomiting, hyperglycemia.

IV Infusion
3 mg initially followed by infusion at 3 mg/hour as necessary.

Drug/Therapy	Indications/Precautions	Adult Dosage
Glycoprotein IIb/IIIa Inhibitors	**Indications** These drugs inhibit the integrin glycoprotein IIb/IIIa receptor in the membrane of platelets, inhibiting platelet aggregation. Indicated for UA/NSTEMI. **Precautions/Contraindications** Active internal bleeding or bleeding disorder in past 30 days, history of intracranial hemorrhage or other bleeding, surgical procedure or trauma within 1 month, platelet count <150 000/mm^3, hypersensitivity and concomitant use of another GP IIb/IIIa inhibitor (also see "ACS: Treatment for UA/NSTEMI").	**Note: Check package insert for current indications, doses, and duration of therapy.** Optimal duration of therapy has not been established. Consultation with expert advised.
Abciximab (ReoPro®)	**Abciximab Indications** FDA-approved for patients with NSTEMI or unstable angina with planned PCI within 24 hours. **Abciximab Precautions/Contraindications** Must use with heparin. Binds irreversibly with platelets. Platelet function recovery requires 48 hours (regeneration). Readministration may cause hypersensitivity reaction.	**Abciximab** • **PCI:** 0.25 mg/kg IV bolus (10 to 60 minutes before procedure), then 0.125 µg/kg per minute (to max of 10 µg/min) IV infusion for 12 hours. • **ACS with planned PCI within 24 hours:** 0.25 mg/kg IV bolus, then 10 µg/min IV infusion for 18 to 24 hours, concluding 1 hour after PCI.

Eptifibatide (Integrilin®)

Eptifibatide Indications
UA/NSTEMI managed medically and patients undergoing PCI.

Actions/Precautions
Platelet function recovers within 4 to 8 hours after discontinuation.

Eptifibatide
- **Medical management:** 180 µg/kg IV bolus over 1 to 2 minutes, then 2 µg/kg per minute IV infusion for 72 to 96 hours.
- **PCI:** 180 µg/kg IV bolus over 1 to 2 minutes, then begin 2 µg/kg per minute IV infusion, then repeat bolus in 10 minutes.
- Maximum dose (121 kg patient) for PCI: 22.6 mg bolus; 15 mg/h infusion. Infusion duration 18 to 24 hours after PCI
- Reduce rate of infusion by 50% if creatinine clearance <50 mL/min.

Tirofiban (Aggrastat®)

Tirofiban Indications
UA/NSTEMI managed medically and patients undergoing PCI.

Actions/Precautions
Platelet function recovers within 4 to 8 hours after discontinuation.

Tirofiban
- **Medical management or PCI:** 0.4 µg/kg per minute IV for 30 minutes, then 0.1 µg/kg per minute IV infusion (for 18 to 24 hours after PCI).
- Reduce rate of infusion by 50% if creatinine clearance <30 mL/min.

Drug/Therapy	Indications/Precautions	Adult Dosage
Heparin Unfractionated (UFH) Concentrations range from 1000 to 40 000 IU/mL	**Indications** • Adjuvant therapy in AMI. • Begin heparin with fibrin-specific lytics (eg, alteplase, reteplase, tenecteplase). **Precautions/Contraindications** • Same contraindications as for fibrinolytic therapy: active bleeding; recent intracranial, intraspinal, or eye surgery; severe hypertension; bleeding disorders; gastrointestinal bleeding. • Doses and laboratory targets appropriate when used with fibrinolytic therapy. • Do not use if platelet count is or falls below <100 000 or with history of heparin-induced thrombocytopenia. For these patients consider direct antithrombins. See bivalirudin at the bottom of this column.	**UFH IV Infusion—STEMI** • Initial bolus 60 IU/kg (maximum bolus: 4000 IU). • Continue 12 IU/kg per hour, round to the nearest 50 IU (maximum: 1000 IU/hour for patients >70 kg). • Adjust to maintain aPTT 1.5 to 2 times the control values (50 to 70 seconds) for 48 hours or until angiography. • Check initial aPTT at 3 hours, then q 6 hours until stable, then daily. • Follow institutional heparin protocol. • Platelet count daily. **UFH IV Infusion—UA/NSTEMI** • Initial bolus 60 IU/kg. Maximum: 4000 IU. • 12 IU/kg per hour. Maximum: 1000 IU/h. • Follow institutional protocol (see Heparin in ACS section).

Heparin
Low Molecular Weight (LMWH)

Indications

For use in acute coronary syndromes, specifically patients with UA/NSTEMI. These drugs inhibit thrombin generation by factor Xa inhibition and also inhibit thrombin indirectly by formation of a complex with antithrombin III. These drugs are **not** neutralized by heparin-binding proteins.

Precautions

- Hemorrhage may complicate any therapy with LMWH. Contraindicated in presence of hypersensitivity to heparin or pork products or history of sensitivity to drug. Use **enoxaparin** with extreme caution in patients with type II heparin-induced thrombocytopenia.
- Adjust dose for renal insufficiency.
- Contraindicated if platelet count <100 000. For these patients consider direct antithrombins:
  - **Bivalirudin** (Angiomax, FDA-approved for ACS patients undergoing PCI): Bolus with 0.1 mg/kg IV, then begin infusion of 0.25 mg/kg per hour.

STEMI Protocol

- Enoxaparin
  - Age <75 years, normal creatinine clearance: initial bolus 30 mg IV with second bolus 15 minutes later of 1 mg/kg SQ, repeat q 12 hours.
  - Age ≥75 years: Eliminate initial IV bolus, give 0.75 mg/kg SQ q 12 hours.
  - If creatinine clearance <30 mL/min, give 1 mg/kg SQ q 24 hours.
- Fondaparinux
  - Initial dose 2.5 mg/kg IV, then give 2.5 mg/kg SQ q 24 hours for up to 8 days.

UA/NSTEMI Protocol

- Enoxaparin: Loading dose 30 mg IV bolus. Maintenance dose 1 mg/kg SQ q 12 hours. If creatinine clearance <30 mL/min, reduce dosing interval to q 24 hours.
- Fondaparinux: 2.5 mg SQ ONCE every 24 hours; avoid if creatinine clearance <30 mL/min.

Heparin Reversal

ICH or life-threatening bleed: Administer protamine, refer to package insert.

Drug/Therapy	Indications/Precautions	Adult Dosage
Ibutilide Intervention of choice is DC cardioversion	**Indications** Treatment of supraventricular arrhythmias, including atrial fibrillation and atrial flutter when duration ≤48 hours. Short duration of action. Effective for the conversion of atrial fibrillation or flutter of relatively brief duration. **Precautions/Contraindications** Contraindication: Do not give to patients with QT_c >440 msec. Ventricular arrhythmias develop in approximately 2% to 5% of patients (polymorphic ventricular tachycardia, including torsades de pointes). *Monitor ECG continuously for arrhythmias during administration and for 4 to 6 hours after administration with defibrillator nearby.* Patients with significantly impaired LV function are at highest risk for arrhythmias.	**Dose for Adults ≥60 kg** 1 mg (10 mL) administered IV (diluted or undiluted) over 10 minutes. A second dose may be administered at the same rate 10 minutes later. **Dose for Adults <60 kg** 0.01 mg/kg initial IV dose.
*Inamrinone Phosphodiesterase enzyme inhibitor *(continued)*	**Indications** Severe congestive heart failure refractory to diuretics, vasodilators, and conventional inotropic agents.	**IV Loading Dose and Infusion** • 0.75 mg/kg (not to exceed 1 mg/kg), given over 2 to 3 minutes. Give loading dose over 10 to 15 minutes with LV dysfunction (eg, postresuscitation).

*Inamrinone *(continued)*

Note: Inamrinone has been replaced by Milrinone in Canada

Precautions
- Do not mix with dextrose solutions or other drugs.
- May cause tachyarrhythmias, hypotension, or thrombocytopenia.
- Can increase myocardial ischemia.

- Follow with infusion of 5 to 15 µg/kg per minute titrated to clinical effect.
- Additional bolus may be given in 30 minutes.
- Requires hemodynamic monitoring.
- Creatinine clearance <10 mL/min: reduce dose 25% to 50%.

Isoproterenol

IV infusion

Indications
- *Use cautiously as temporizing measure if external pacer is not available* for treatment of symptomatic bradycardia.
- Refractory torsades de pointes unresponsive to magnesium sulfate.
- *Temporary* control of bradycardia in heart transplant patients (denervated heart unresponsive to atropine).
- Poisoning from β-blockers.

Precautions
- Do not use for treatment of cardiac arrest.
- Increases myocardial oxygen requirements, which may increase myocardial ischemia.
- Do not give with epinephrine; can cause VF/VT.
- Do not give to patients with poison/drug-induced shock (except for β-blocker poisoning).
- May use higher doses for β-blocker poisoning.

IV Administration
- Infuse at 2 to 10 µg/min.
- Titrate to adequate heart rate.
- In torsades de pointes titrate to increase heart rate until VT is suppressed.

Drug/Therapy	Indications/Precautions	Adult Dosage
Lidocaine Can be given via endotracheal tube	**Indications** • Alternative to amiodarone in cardiac arrest from VF/VT. • Stable monomorphic VT with preserved ventricular function. • Stable polymorphic VT with normal baseline QT interval and preserved LV function when ischemia is treated and electrolyte balance is corrected. • Can be used for stable polymorphic VT with baseline QT-interval prolongation if torsades suspected. **Precautions/Contraindications** • **Contraindication:** *Prophylactic* use in AMI is contraindicated. • Reduce maintenance dose (not loading dose) in presence of impaired liver function or left ventricular dysfunction. • Discontinue infusion immediately if signs of toxicity develop.	**Cardiac Arrest From VF/VT** • Initial dose: 1 to 1.5 mg/kg IV/IO. • For refractory VF may give additional 0.5 to 0.75 mg/kg IV push, repeat in 5 to 10 minutes; maximum 3 doses or total of 3 mg/kg. • Endotracheal administration: 2 to 4 mg/kg. **Perfusing Arrhythmia** For stable VT, wide-complex tachycardia of uncertain type, significant ectopy: • Doses ranging from 0.5 to 0.75 mg/kg and up to 1 to 1.5 mg/kg may be used. • Repeat 0.5 to 0.75 mg/kg every 5 to 10 minutes: maximum total dose: 3 mg/kg. **Maintenance Infusion** 1 to 4 mg/min (30 to 50 µg/kg per minute); can dilute in D_5W, $D_{10}W$, or NS.

Magnesium Sulfate

Indications
- Recommended for use in cardiac arrest only if torsades de pointes or suspected hypomagnesemia is present.
- Life-threatening ventricular arrhythmias due to digitalis toxicity.
- Routine administration in hospitalized patients with AMI is **not** recommended.

Precautions
- Occasional fall in blood pressure with rapid administration.
- Use with caution if renal failure is present.

Cardiac Arrest
(Due to Hypomagnesemia or Torsades de Pointes)
1 to 2 g (2 to 4 mL of a 50% solution) diluted in 10 mL of D_5W IV/IO over 5 to 20 minutes.

Torsades de Pointes With a Pulse or AMI With Hypomagnesemia
- Loading dose of 1 to 2 g mixed in 50 to 100 mL of D_5W, over 5 to 60 minutes IV.
- Follow with 0.5 to 1 g/h IV (titrate to control torsades).

Mannitol

Strengths: 5%, 10%, 15%, 20%, and 25%

Indications
Increased intracranial pressure in management of neurologic emergencies.

Precautions
- Monitor fluid status and serum osmolality (not to exceed 310 mOsm/kg).
- Caution in renal failure because fluid overload may result.

IV Administration
- Administer 0.5 to 1 g/kg over 5 to 10 minutes through in-line filter.
- Additional doses of 0.25 to 2 g/kg can be given every 4 to 6 hours as needed.
- Use with support of oxygenation and ventilation.

Advanced Cardiovascular Life Support Drugs and Electrical Therapy

ACLS

Drug/Therapy	Indications/Precautions	Adult Dosage
Milrinone Shorter half-life than inamrinone	**Indications** Myocardial dysfunction and increased systemic or pulmonary vascular resistance, including • Congestive heart failure in postoperative cardiovascular surgical patients • Shock with high systemic vascular resistance **Precautions** May produce nausea, vomiting, hypotension, particularly in volume-depleted patients. Shorter half-life and less effect on platelets but more risk for ventricular arrhythmia than inamrinone. Drug may accumulate in renal failure and in patients with low cardiac output; reduce dose in renal failure.	**Loading Dose** 50 µg/kg over 10 minutes IV loading dose. **Intravenous Infusion** • 0.375 to 0.75 µg/kg per minute for 2 to 3 days. • Hemodynamic monitoring required. • Reduce dose in renal impairment.
Morphine Sulfate *(continued)*	**Indications** • Chest pain with ACS unresponsive to nitrates. • Acute cardiogenic pulmonary edema (if blood pressure is adequate).	**IV Administration** • STEMI: Give 2 to 4 mg IV. May give additional doses of 2 to 8 mg IV at 5- to 15-minute intervals. Analgesic of choice.

Morphine Sulfate *(continued)*	**Precautions** • Administer slowly and titrate to effect. • May cause respiratory depression. • Causes hypotension in volume-depleted patients. • Use with caution in right ventricular infarction. • May reverse with naloxone (0.4 to 2 mg IV).	• UA/NSTEMI: Give 1 to 5 mg IV only if symptoms not relieved by nitrates or if symptoms recur.
Naloxone Hydrochloride	**Indications** Respiratory and neurologic depression due to opiate intoxication unresponsive to O_2 and support of ventilation. **Precautions** • May cause opiate withdrawal. • Half-life shorter than narcotics, repeat dosing may be needed. • Monitor for recurrent respiratory depression. • Rare anaphylactic reactions have been reported. • Assist ventilation before naloxone administration, avoid sympathetic stimulation. • Avoid in meperidine-induced seizures.	**Administration** • Typical dose 0.4 to 2 mg, titrate until ventilation adequate. • Use higher doses for complete narcotic reversal. • Can administer up to 6 to 10 mg over short period (<10 minutes). • IM/SQ 0.4 to 0.8 mg • For chronic opioid-addicted patients, use smaller dose and titrate slowly. • Can be given by endotracheal route if IV/IO access not available (other routes preferred).

Drug/Therapy	Indications/Precautions	Adult Dosage

Nitroglycerin
 	
Available in IV form, sublingual tablets, and aerosol spray
	Indications
	• Initial antianginal for suspected ischemic pain.
	• For initial 24 to 48 hours in patients with *AMI and CHF*, large anterior wall infarction, persistent or recurrent ischemia, or hypertension.
	• Continued use (beyond 48 hours) for patients with recurrent angina or persistent pulmonary congestion (nitrate-free interval recommended).
	• Hypertensive urgency with ACS.
	
	Contraindications
	• Hypotension (SBP <90 mm Hg or more than 30 mm Hg below baseline).
	• Severe bradycardia (<50 per minute) or tachycardia (>100 per minute).
	• RV infarction.
	• Use of phosphodiesterase inhibitors for erectile dysfunction (eg, sildenafil and vardenafil within 24 hours; tadalafil within 48 hours). ↓
		IV Administration
		• IV bolus: 12.5 to 25 µg (if no SL or spray given).
		• Infusion: Begin at 10 µg/min. Titrate to effect, increase by 10 µg/min every 3 to 5 minutes until desired effect. Ceiling dose of 200 µg/min commonly used.
		  — Route of choice for emergencies.
		  — Use appropriate IV sets provided by pharmaceutical companies.
		• Dilute in D_5W or NS.
		
		Sublingual Route
		1 tablet (0.3 to 0.4 mg), repeated for total of 3 doses at 5-minute intervals.
		
		Aerosol Spray
		1 to 2 sprays for 0.5 to 1 second at 5-minute intervals (provides 0.4 mg per dose). Maximum 3 sprays within 15 minutes. ↓

(continued)

Nitroglycerin *(continued)*	**Precautions** • Generally, with evidence of AMI and normotension, do not reduce systolic BP to <110 mm Hg. If patient is hypertensive, do not decrease mean arterial pressure (MAP) by more than 25% (from initial MAP). • Do not mix with other drugs. • Patient should sit or lie down when receiving this medication. • Do not shake aerosol spray because this affects metered dose.	**Note:** Patients should be instructed to contact EMS if pain is unrelieved or increasing after one tablet or sublingual spray.
Nitroprusside (Sodium Nitroprusside)	**Indications** • Hypertensive crisis. • To reduce afterload in heart failure and acute pulmonary edema. • To reduce afterload in acute mitral or aortic valve regurgitation. **Precautions** • May cause hypotension, thiocyanate toxicity, and CO_2 retention. • May reverse hypoxic pulmonary vasoconstriction in patients with pulmonary disease, exacerbating intrapulmonary shunting, resulting in hypoxemia. • Other side effects include headaches, nausea, vomiting, and abdominal cramps. • Caution with phosphodiesterase inhibitors (eg, sildenafil).	**IV Administration** • Add 50 or 100 mg to 250 mL D_5W. (Refer to your institutional pharmacy policy.) • Begin at 0.1 µg/kg per minute and titrate upward every 3 to 5 minutes to desired effect (usually up to 5 µg/kg per minute, but higher doses up to 10 µg/kg may be needed). • Use with an infusion pump; use hemodynamic monitoring for optimal safety. • Action occurs within 1 to 2 minutes. • Light-sensitive; cover drug reservoir and tubing with opaque material.

Drug/Therapy	Indications/Precautions	Adult Dosage
Norepinephrine	**Indications** • Severe cardiogenic shock and hemodynamically significant hypotension (systolic blood pressure <70 mm Hg) with low total peripheral resistance. • Agent of last resort for management of ischemic heart disease and shock. **Precautions** • Increases myocardial oxygen requirements, raises blood pressure and heart rate. • May induce arrhythmias. Use with caution in patients with acute ischemia; monitor cardiac output. • Extravasation causes tissue necrosis. • If extravasation occurs, administer phentolamine 5 to 10 mg in 10 to 15 mL saline solution, infiltrate into area.	**IV Administration (Only Route)** • 0.5 to 1 µg/min titrated to improve blood pressure (up to 30 µg/min). • Add 4 mg of norepinephrine or 8 mg of norepinephrine bitartrate to 250 mL of D_5W or D_5NS, but not NS alone. • Do not administer in same IV line as alkaline solutions. • Poison/drug-induced hypotension may require higher doses to achieve adequate perfusion.

Oxygen

Delivered from portable tanks or installed, wall-mounted sources through delivery devices

Indications

- Any suspected cardiopulmonary emergency.
- Complaints of shortness of breath and suspected ischemic pain.
- ACS: administer to all patients for first 6 hours. Continue if pulmonary congestion, ongoing ischemia, or oxygen saturation is <90%.
- For patients with suspected stroke and hypoxemia or unknown oxyhemoglobin saturation. May consider administration to patients who are not hypoxemic.

Precautions

- Observe closely when using with pulmonary patients known to be dependent on hypoxic respiratory drive (very rare).
- Pulse oximetry may be inaccurate in low cardiac output states, with vasoconstriction, or with carbon monoxide exposure.

Device	Flow Rate	O_2 (%)
Nasal cannula	1-6 L/min	21-44
Venturi mask	4-12 L/min	24-50
Partial rebreather mask	6-10 L/min	35-60
Nonrebreather O_2 mask with reservoir	6-15 L/min	60-100
Bag-mask with nonrebreather "tail"	15 L/min	95-100

Note: Pulse oximetry provides a useful method of titrating oxygen administration to maintain physiologic oxygen saturation (see Precautions).

Drug/Therapy	Indications/Precautions	Adult Dosage

Procainamide	**Indications**
	• Useful for treatment of a wide variety of arrhythmias, including stable monomorphic VT with normal QT interval and preserved LV function.
	• May use for treatment of re-entry SVT uncontrolled by adenosine and vagal maneuvers if blood pressure stable.
	• Stable wide-complex tachycardia of unknown origin.
	• Atrial fibrillation with rapid rate in Wolff-Parkinson-White syndrome.
	
	Precautions
	• If cardiac or renal dysfunction is present, reduce maximum total dose to 12 mg/kg and maintenance infusion to 1 to 2 mg/min.
	• Proarrhythmic, especially in setting of AMI, hypokalemia, or hypomagnesemia.
	• May induce hypotension in patients with impaired LV function.
	• Use with caution with other drugs that prolong QT interval. Expert consultation advised.
		Recurrent VF/VT
		• 20 mg/min IV infusion (maximum total dose: 17 mg/kg).
		• In urgent situations, up to 50 mg/min may be administered to total dose of 17 mg/kg.
		
		Other Indications
		• 20 mg/min IV infusion until one of the following occurs:
		  — Arrhythmia suppression
		  — Hypotension
		  — QRS widens by >50%
		  — Total dose of 17 mg/kg is given
		• Use in cardiac arrest limited by need for slow infusion and uncertain efficacy.
		
		Maintenance Infusion
		1 to 4 mg/min (dilute in D_5W or NS). Reduce dose in presence of renal insufficiency.

Sodium Bicarbonate

Indications

Specific indications for bicarbonate use are as follows:

- Known preexisting hyperkalemia.
- Known preexisting bicarbonate-responsive acidosis; eg, diabetic ketoacidosis or overdose of tricyclic antidepressant, aspirin, cocaine, or diphenhydramine.
- Prolonged resuscitation with effective ventilation; upon return of spontaneous circulation after long arrest interval.
- Not useful or effective in hypercarbic acidosis (eg, cardiac arrest and CPR without intubation).

Precautions

- Adequate ventilation and CPR, not bicarbonate, are the major "buffer agents" in cardiac arrest.
- Not recommended for routine use in cardiac arrest patients.

IV Administration

- 1 mEq/kg IV bolus.
- If rapidly available, use arterial blood gas analysis to guide bicarbonate therapy (calculated base deficits or bicarbonate concentration). ABG results not reliable indicators of acidosis during cardiac arrest.

Drug/Therapy	Indications/Precautions	Adult Dosage
Sotalol *(IV form not approved for use in United States)* Not a first-line antiarrhythmic Seek expert consultation	**Indications** In the United States, oral form is approved for treatment of ventricular and atrial arrhythmias. Outside the United States, used for treatment of supraventricular arrhythmias and ventricular arrhythmias in patients without structural heart disease. **Precautions/Contraindications** • Should be avoided in patients with poor perfusion because of significant negative inotropic effects. ***Must be infused slowly.*** • Adverse effects include bradycardia, hypotension, and arrhythmias (torsades de pointes). • Use with caution with other drugs that prolong QT interval (eg, procainamide, amiodarone).	**IV Administration** • 1 to 1.5 mg/kg body weight, then infused at rate of 10 mg/min. • ***Must be infused slowly.*** • Reduce dose with renal impairment.
Thrombolytic Agents *(see **Fibrinolytic Agents**)*		

Transcutaneous Pacing

External pacemakers have either *fixed* rates (nondemand or asynchronous mode) or *demand* rates (range: 30 to 180 per minute).

Current outputs range from 0 to 200 mA.

Indications

- Hemodynamically unstable or symptomatic bradycardia (eg, blood pressure changes, altered mental status, angina, pulmonary edema).
- Pacing readiness in setting of AMI, as follows:
  - Symptomatic sinus node dysfunction.
  - Type II second-degree heart block.
  - Third-degree heart block.
  - New left, right, or alternating BBB or bifascicular block.
- Bradycardia with symptomatic ventricular escape rhythms.
- Overdrive pacing of tachycardias refractory to drug therapy or electrical cardioversion.
- Not recommended for bradyasystolic cardiac arrest.

Precautions

- Contraindicated in severe hypothermia or prolonged bradyasystolic cardiac arrest.
- Conscious patients may require analgesia for discomfort.
- Avoid using carotid pulse to confirm mechanical capture. Electrical stimulation causes muscular jerking that may mimic carotid pulse.

Technique

- Place pacing electrodes on chest per package instructions.
- Turn the pacer ON.
- Set demand rate to approximately 80 per minute.
- Set current (mA) output as follows for *bradycardia:* Increase milliamperes from minimum setting until consistent capture is achieved (characterized by a widening QRS and a broad T wave after each pacer spike). Then add 2 mA for safety margin.

Drug/Therapy	Indications/Precautions	Adult Dosage
Vasopressin	**Indications** • May be used as an alternative pressor to epinephrine in the treatment of adult shock-refractory VF. • May be useful alternative to epinephrine in asystole, PEA. • May be useful for hemodynamic support in vasodilatory shock (eg, septic shock). **Precautions/Contraindications** • Potent peripheral vasoconstrictor. Increased peripheral vascular resistance may provoke cardiac ischemia and angina. • Not recommended for responsive patients with coronary artery disease.	**IV Administration** **One dose for cardiac arrest:** 40 U IV/IO push may replace either first or second dose of epinephrine. Epinephrine can be administerd every 3 to 5 minutes during cardiac arrest. Vasopressin may be given by the endotracheal route, but at this time there is insufficient evidence to recommend a specific dose.
Verapamil	**Indications** • Alternative drug (after adenosine) to terminate re-entry SVT with narrow QRS complex and adequate blood pressure and *preserved LV function.* • May control ventricular response in patients with atrial fibrillation, flutter, or multifocal atrial tachycardia. **Precautions** • Give *only* to patients with narrow-complex reentry SVT or known supraventricular arrhythmias.	**IV Administration** • **First dose:** 2.5 to 5 mg IV bolus over 2 minutes (over 3 minutes in older patients). • **Second dose:** 5 to 10 mg, if needed, every 15 to 30 minutes. Maximum dose: 20 mg. • **Alternative:** 5 mg bolus every 15 minutes to total dose of 30 mg.

(continued) ↓

Verapamil
(continued)

- Do not use for wide-QRS tachycardias of uncertain origin, and avoid use for Wolff-Parkinson-White syndrome and atrial fibrillation, sick sinus syndrome, or second- or third-degree AV block without pacemaker.
- May decrease myocardial contractility and can produce peripheral vasodilation and hypotension. IV calcium may restore blood pressure in toxic cases.
- Concurrent IV administration with IV β-blockers may produce severe hypotension. Use with extreme caution in patients receiving oral β-blockers.

Useful Calculations and Formulae		
Calculation	**Formula**	**Comments**
Anion gap (serum concentration in mEq/L)	$[Na^+] - ([Cl^-] + [HCO_3^-])$	Normal range: 10 to 15 mEq/L. A gap >15 suggests metabolic acidosis.
Osmolal gap	$Osmolality_{measured} - Osmolality_{calculated}$ Normal = <10	Osmolal gap normally <10. If osmolal gap is >10, suspect unknown osmotically active substances.
Calculated osmolality (in mOsm/L)	$(2 \times [Na^+]) + ([Glucose] \div 18) + ([BUN] \div 2.8)$	Simplified to give *effective* osmolality. Normal = 272 to 300 mOsm/L
Total free water deficit (in L)	$\dfrac{([Na^+]_{measured} - 140) \times TBW}{140}$ $TBW_{in\ L} = (0.6_{men}\ or\ 0.5_{women}) \times Weight_{in\ kg}$	Use to calculate quantity of water needed to correct water deficit in hypernatremia.

Sodium deficit (in total mEq)	$([Na^+]_{desired} - [Na^+]_{measured}) \times TBW_{in\ L}$ $TBW_{in\ L} = (0.6_{men}\ or\ 0.5_{women}) \times Weight_{in\ kg}$	Use to calculate sodium deficit that is partially treated with 3% saline in severe hyponatremia (3% saline contains 513 mEq sodium per liter). Plan to raise serum sodium: • Asymptomatic: 0.5 mEq/L per hour • Neurologic symptoms: 1 mEq/L per hour until symptoms controlled • Seizures: 2 to 4 mEq/L per hour until seizures are controlled
Determination of *predicted* pH	$(40 - P_{CO_2}) \times 0.008 = \pm\Delta$ in pH from 7.4	For every 1 mm Hg uncompensated change in P_{CO_2} from 40, pH will change by 0.008. Measured pH less than predicted pH: metabolic acidosis is present. Measured pH greater than predicted pH: metabolic alkalosis is present.

Emergency Treatments and Treatment Sequence for Hyperkalemia

Therapy	Dose	Effect Mechanism	Onset of Effect	Duration of Effect
Calcium chloride	■ 5 to 10 mL IV 10% solution (500 to 1000 mg)	■ Antagonism of toxic effects of hyperkalemia at cell membrane	■ 1 to 3 min	■ 30 to 60 min
Sodium bicarbonate	■ Begin with 1 ampule; give up to 1 mEq/kg ■ Repeat in 15 min ■ Then give 2 ampules (100 mEq) in 1 L D_5W IV PRN over next 1 to 2 hours	■ Redistribution: intracellular shift	■ 5 to 10 min	■ 1 to 2 h
Insulin plus glucose (use 2 U insulin per 5 g glucose)	■ 10 U regular insulin IV plus 1 ampule (50 mL) D_{50} (25 g)	■ Redistribution: intracellular shift	■ 30 min	■ 4 to 6 h

	■ Then give 10 to 20 U regular insulin and 500 mL $D_{10}W$ IV over 1 h PRN			
Nebulized albuterol	■ 10 to 20 mg over 15 min ■ May repeat	■ Redistribution: intracellular shift	■ 15 min	■ 15 to 90 min
Diuresis with furosemide	■ 40 to 80 mg IV bolus	■ Removal from body	■ At start of diuresis	■ Until end of diuresis
Cation-exchange resin (Kayexalate)	■ 15 to 50 g PO or PR plus sorbitol	■ Removal from body	■ 1 to 2 h	■ 4 to 6 h
Peritoneal or hemodialysis	■ Per institutional protocol	■ Removal from body	■ At start of dialysis	■ Until end of dialysis

Potentially Toxic Drugs: by Type of Agent	Cardiopulmonary Signs* of Toxicity	Therapy to Consider†
Stimulants (sympathomimetics) • Amphetamines • Methamphetamines • Cocaine • Phencyclidine (PCP) • Ephedrine	• Tachycardia • Supraventricular arrhythmias • Ventricular arrhythmias • Impaired conduction • Hypertensive crises • Acute coronary syndromes • Shock • Cardiac arrest	• Benzodiazepines • Lidocaine • Sodium bicarbonate (for cocaine-related ventricular arrhythmias) • Nitroglycerin • Nitroprusside • Reperfusion strategy based on cardiac catheterization data • Phentolamine (α_1-adrenergic blocker) • β-blockers relatively contraindicated (do not use propranolol for cocaine intoxication)
Calcium channel blockers • Verapamil • Nifedipine (and other dihydropyridines) • Diltiazem	• Bradycardia • Impaired conduction • Shock • Cardiac arrest	• NS boluses (0.5 to 1 L) • Epinephrine IV; or other α/β-agonists • Pacemakers • Circulatory assist devices? • Calcium infusions • Glucose/insulin infusion? • Glucagon

β-Blockers • Atenolol • Metoprolol • Propranolol • Sotalol	• Bradycardia • Impaired conduction • Shock • Cardiac arrest	• NS boluses (0.5 to 1 L) • Epinephrine IV; or other α/β-agonists • Pacemakers • Circulatory assist devices? • Calcium infusions? • Glucose/insulin infusion? • Glucagon
Tricyclic antidepressants • Amitriptyline • Desipramine • Nortriptyline • Imipramine	• Tachycardia • Bradycardia • Ventricular arrhythmias • Impaired conduction • Shock • Cardiac arrest	• Sodium bicarbonate • Hyperventilation • NS boluses (0.5 to 1 L) • Magnesium sulfate • Lidocaine • Epinephrine IV; or other α/β-agonists
Cardiac glycosides • Digoxin • Digitoxin • Foxglove • Oleander	• Bradycardia • Supraventricular arrhythmias • Ventricular arrhythmias • Impaired conduction • Shock • Cardiac arrest	• Restore total body K^+, Mg^{++} • Restore intravascular volume • Digoxin-specific antibodies (Fab fragments: *Digibind* or *DigiFab*) • Atropine • Pacemakers (use caution and monitor for ventricular arrhythmias) • Lidocaine • Phenytoin?

*Unless stated otherwise, listed alterations in vital signs (bradycardia, tachycardia, tachypnea) are "hemodynamically significant."
†Specific *therapy to consider* should be based on specific indications. Therapies followed by "?" are *Class Indeterminate*.

Potentially Toxic Drugs: by Type of Agent	Cardiopulmonary Signs* of Toxicity	Therapy to Consider†
Anticholinergics • Diphenhydramine • Doxylamine	• Tachycardia • Supraventricular arrhythmias • Ventricular arrhythmias • Impaired conduction • Shock, cardiac arrest	• Physostigmine
Cholinergics • Carbamates • Nerve agents • Organophosphates	• Bradycardia • Ventricular arrhythmias • Impaired conduction, shock • Pulmonary edema • Bronchospasm • Cardiac arrest	• Atropine • Decontamination • Pralidoxime • Obidoxime
Opioids • Heroin • Fentanyl • Methadone • Morphine	• Hypoventilation (slow and shallow respirations, apnea) • Bradycardia • Hypotension • Miosis (pupil constriction)	• Assisted ventilation • Naloxone • Tracheal intubation • Nalmefene

Isoniazid	• Lactic acidosis with/without seizures • Tachycardia or bradycardia • Shock, cardiac arrest	• Pyridoxine (vitamin B_6)—large doses may be needed (eg, 1 g pyridoxine/g of ingested isoniazid)
Sodium channel blockers (Class I$_{vw}$ antiarrhythmics) • Procainamide • Disopyramide • Lidocaine • Propafenone • Flecainide	• Bradycardia • Ventricular arrhythmias • Impaired conduction • Seizures • Shock, cardiac arrest	• Sodium bicarbonate • Pacemakers • α- and β-agonist • Lidocaine (except for lidocaine toxicity) • Hypertonic saline

*Unless stated otherwise, listed alterations in vital signs (bradycardia, tachycardia, tachypnea) are "hemodynamically significant."
†Specific *therapy to consider* should be based on specific indications. Therapies followed by "?" are *Class Indeterminate*.

Drug-Induced Cardiovascular Emergency or Altered Vital Signs*	Therapies to Consider†	Contraindicated Interventions (or Use With Caution)
Bradycardia	• Pacemaker (transcutaneous or transvenous) • Toxic drug—*calcium channel blocker*: epinephrine, calcium salt? glucose/insulin? glucagon? NS (if hypotensive) • Toxic drug—β-blocker: NS, epinephrine, calcium salt? glucose/insulin? glucagon?	• Atropine (seldom helpful except for cholinesterase inhibitor poisonings) • Isoproterenol if hypotensive • Prophylactic transvenous pacing
Tachycardia	• Toxic drug—*sympathomimetics*: benzodiazepines, lidocaine, sodium bicarbonate, nitroglycerin, nitroprusside, labetalol • Toxic drug—*tricyclic antidepressants*: sodium bicarbonate, hyperventilation, NS, magnesium sulfate, lidocaine • Toxic drug—*anticholinergics*: physostigmine	• β-blockers (not generally useful in drug-induced tachycardia) • Do not use propranolol for cocaine intoxication • Cardioversion (rarely indicated) • Adenosine (rarely indicated) • Calcium channel blockers (rarely indicated) • Physostigmine (if TCA overdose)
Impaired conduction/ventricular arrhythmias	• Sodium bicarbonate • Lidocaine	• If TCA overdose: amiodarone or type I_{vw} antiarrhythmics (eg, procainamide)
Hypertensive emergencies	• Toxic drug—*sympathomimetics*: benzodiazepines, lidocaine, sodium bicarbonate, nitroglycerin, nitroprusside, phentolamine	• β-blockers

Acute coronary syndrome	• Benzodiazepines • Lidocaine • Sodium bicarbonate • Nitroglycerin • Aspirin, heparin • Base reperfusion strategy on cardiac catheterization data	• β-blockers
Shock	• Toxic drug—*calcium channel blocker:* NS, epinephrine, norepinephrine, dopamine, calcium salt? glucose/insulin? glucagon? • Toxic drug—*β-blocker:* NS, epinephrine, norepinephrine, dopamine, calcium salt? glucose/insulin? glucagon? • If refractory to *maximal* medical therapy: consider circulatory assist devices	• Isoproterenol • Avoid calcium salts if digoxin toxicity is suspected
Acute cholinergic syndrome	• Atropine • Pralidoxime/obidoxime	• Succinylcholine
Acute anticholinergic syndrome	• Benzodiazepine • Physostigmine (not for TCA overdose)	• Antipsychotics • Other anticholinergic agents
Opioid poisoning	• Assisted ventilation • Naloxone • Tracheal intubation	• Do not use naloxone for meperidine-induced seizures

*Unless stated otherwise, listed alterations of vital signs (bradycardia, tachycardia, tachypnea) are "hemodynamically significant."
Therapies to consider should be based on specific indications.
†NS indicates normal saline; TCA, tricyclic antidepressant

Pre-event Equipment Checklist for Endotracheal Intubation
Equipment and Drugs Recommended for Endotracheal Intubation

Yes?	No?	Equipment
		Cardiac monitor
		Automatic blood pressure cuff
		Intravenous infusion equipment
		Oxygen supply, equipment for connections to airway adjunct device
		Esophageal detector device (aspiration technique)
		Exhaled CO_2 detector device: capnometry (qualitative) **or** Exhaled CO_2 measuring device: capnography (continuous, quantitative)
		Pulse oximeter
		Suction device and suction catheter (confirm working; catheter near patient head)
		Bag-mask connected to high-flow oxygen source
		Endotracheal tubes, proper size (all sizes should be available for emergent use; typically the size above and below anticipated size for the patient should be within reach during the attempt)

		Endotracheal tube stylet
		Laryngoscope blade (curved and straight available) with working bulb
		Laryngoscope handle with connector and battery
		Backup light source (another laryngoscope handle and blade)
		5- to 10-mL syringe to test-inflate endotracheal tube balloon (attached to pilot balloon)
		Premedication agents: lidocaine, opioids (such as fentanyl), atropine, and defasciculating agents
		Analgesic agents: opioids
		Sedative/anesthetic agents: etomidate, propofol, methohexital, thiopental, midazolam, ketamine
		Paralytic agents: succinylcholine, vecuronium, pancuronium, rocuronium
		Commercial endotracheal tube holder
		Restraints for patient's hands if awake
		Container for patient's dentures if needed
		Towel or pad to place under patient's head (to align airway)
		Specialty equipment as needed for difficult airway management or anticipated complications.

Modify where appropriate.

Rapid Sequence Intubation Protocol

Rapid Sequence Intubation Protocol

Steps	Details
Preoxygenate	1. Preoxygenate with 100% oxygen by mask. If ventilatory assistance is necessary, ventilate gently. Apply cricoid pressure if victim is unconscious.
Premedicate	2. Premedicate as appropriate; then WAIT 3 MINUTES after drug administration. • *Fentanyl:* 2 to 3 μg/kg given at a rate of 1 to 2 μg/kg per minute IV for analgesia in awake patients • *Atropine:* 0.02 mg/kg IV push (minimum dose of 0.1 mg recommended) • *Lidocaine:* 1.5 to 2 mg/kg IV over 30 to 60 seconds
Paralyze after sedation	3. Induce anesthesia with one of these agents: thiopental, methohexital, fentanyl, ketamine, etomidate, or propofol. 4. Give succinylcholine 1.5 mg/kg IV push. • Defasciculating agent (optional, see "Sedation" below) 5. Assess for apnea, jaw relaxation, decreased resistance to bag-mask ventilations (patient sufficiently relaxed to proceed with intubation). 6. Apply cricoid pressure; WAIT 30 SECONDS.
Placement: performance	7. Perform endotracheal intubation. If unable to intubate within 20 seconds, stop attempt. Ventilate with bag-mask for 30 to 60 seconds. Use pulse oximetry as a guide. Reattempt intubation. 8. Treat bradycardia during intubation with atropine 0.5 mg IV push. • Inflate balloon cuff when ET is in place.
Placement: exam confirmation	9. Perform exam *confirmation* of ET placement: • By direct visualization of ET passing through vocal cords • By chest rise/fall with each ventilation (bilateral) • By 5-point auscultation: anterior chest L and R, midaxillary line L and R, and over the epigastrium. (Listen for air entering the stomach when bag is squeezed. Look for tube condensation.)
Placement: device confirmation	10. Perform *device confirmation* of ET placement: • Cardiac arrest : use esophageal detector device (EDD). • Perfusing rhythm: use end-tidal CO_2 detection. Can use EDD or both. • Monitor O_2 saturation and end-tidal CO_2 levels (capnometry or capnography).
Placement: prevent dislodgment	11. Secure ET with commercial ET holder (preferred). • Alternatively, secure with an adhesive tape/cloth cord technique. • In out-of-hospital setting with the prospect of patient movement, immobilize cervical spine with cervical collar or backboard or both.

Sedation: Sedative and Induction Agents

Sedative	Dosage IV Push	Onset	Duration
Etomidate	0.2 to 0.6 mg/kg	60 seconds	3 to 5 minutes
Fentanyl	*Induction:* 2 to 10 µg/kg *Sedation (titrate):* 3 µg/kg	60 seconds	30 to 60 minutes
Ketamine	2 mg/kg	30 to 60 seconds	15 minutes
Midazolam	*Induction:* 0.15 to 0.30 mg/kg *Sedation (titrate):* 0.02 to 0.04 mg/kg	2 minutes	1 to 2 hours
Propofol	2 to 2.5 mg/kg	40 seconds	3 to 5 minutes
Thiopental	3 to 5 mg/kg	20 to 40 seconds	5 to 10 minutes

Neuromuscular Blocking Agents Used in Tracheal Intubation During Cardiac Arrest

Drug	Dose*	Route	Duration of Paralysis	Side Effects	Comments
Succinylcholine (Anectine)	1 to 2 mg/kg IV; 2 to 4 mg/kg IM	IV, IM†	3-5 min	Muscle fasciculations Rise in intraocular, intragastric, intracranial pressure Life-threatening high level of potassium Hypertension	Depolarizing muscle relaxant Rapid onset; short duration of action Renal failure, burns, high potassium level are contraindications Consider defasciculation with nondepolarizing agent Do not use for maintenance of paralysis
Vecuronium (Norcuron)	0.1-0.2 mg/kg	IV	30-60 min	Minimal cardiovascular side effects	Nondepolarizing agent Onset of action: 2-3 min
Rocuronium (Zemuron)	0.6-1.2 mg/kg	IV	40+ min	Minimal cardiovascular side effects	Nondepolarizing agent Rapid-action onset like succinylcholine

*Doses shown are guidelines only.
†Actual dosing may vary depending on patient's clinical status.

Newborn Resuscitation

Ideally, newborn resuscitation takes place in the delivery room or the neonatal intensive care unit, with trained personnel and appropriate equipment readily available. This form of resuscitation is taught in the **Neonatal Resuscitation Program (NRP)** offered by the American Academy of Pediatrics and the AHA. These pages provide information about initial assessment of the newborn and initial stabilization priorities. *Ensuring adequate ventilation of the baby's lungs is the most important and effective action in neonatal resuscitation.*

Initial Assessment and Stabilization

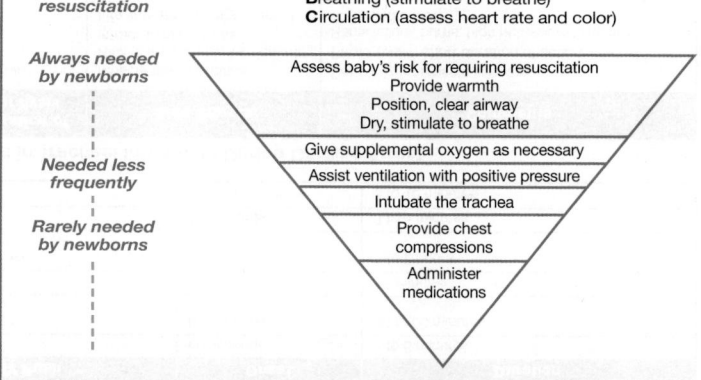

ABCs of resuscitation

Airway (position and clear)
Breathing (stimulate to breathe)
Circulation (assess heart rate and color)

Always needed by newborns

Assess baby's risk for requiring resuscitation
Provide warmth
Position, clear airway
Dry, stimulate to breathe

Needed less frequently

Give supplemental oxygen as necessary

Assist ventilation with positive pressure

Intubate the trachea

Rarely needed by newborns

Provide chest compressions

Administer medications

A majority of newborns respond to simple measures. The inverted pyramid reflects relative frequencies of resuscitative efforts for a newborn who does not have meconium-stained amniotic fluid.

Term Newborn Vital Signs

Heart rate (awake): 100 to 180/min
Respiratory rate: 30 to 60 breaths/min
Systolic blood pressure: 55 to 90 mm Hg
Diastolic blood pressure: 26 to 55 mm Hg

Reproduced from Zubrow AB, Hulman S, Kushner H, Falkner B. Determinants of blood pressure in infants admitted to neonatal intensive care units: a prospective multicenter study. Philadelphia Neonatal Blood Pressure Study Group. *J Perinatol.* 1995;15:470-479.

Apgar Score

Sign	0	1	2
Color	Blue or pale	Pink body with blue extremities (acrocyanotic)	Completely pink
Heart rate	Absent	Slow (<100/min)	> 100/min
Reflex irritability (to a catheter in the nares, tactile stimulation)	No response	Grimace	Cry or active withdrawal
Muscle tone	Limp	Some flexion	Active motion
Respiration	Absent	Weak cry, hypoventilation	Good, crying

Reproduced with minor modification from Kattwinkel J, ed. *Neonatal Resuscitation Textbook,* 5th edition. Elk Grove Villiage, Ill, American Academy of Pediatrics and American Heart Association; 2006:1-28.

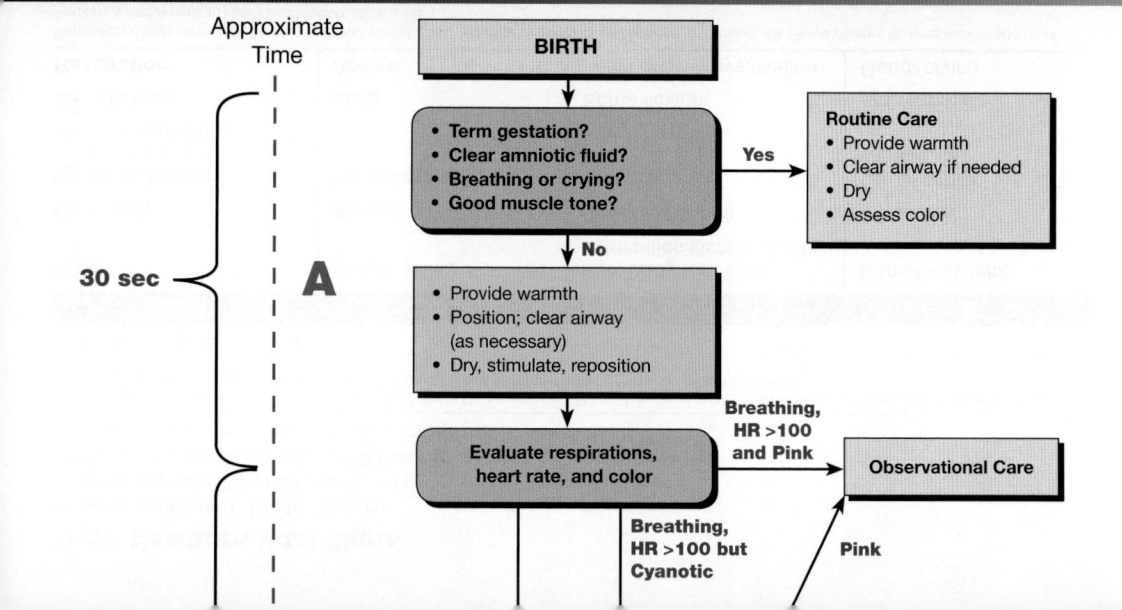

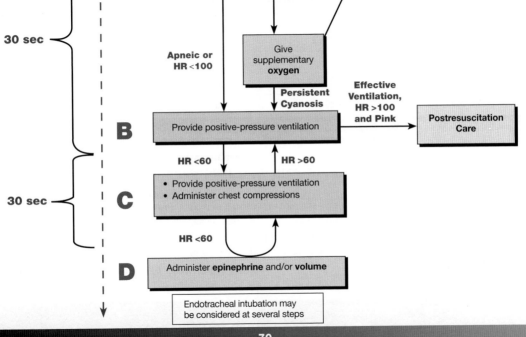

30 sec

Apneic or
HR <100

Give
supplementary **oxygen**

Persistent
Cyanosis

Effective
Ventilation,
HR >100
and Pink

B Provide positive-pressure ventilation → Postresuscitation Care

HR <60   HR >60

C
- Provide positive-pressure ventilation
- Administer chest compressions

30 sec

HR <60

D Administer **epinephrine** and/or **volume**

Endotracheal intubation may
be considered at several steps

Initial Cardiopulmonary Resuscitation

Ventilation rate: 40 to 60/min when performed *without* compressions.

Compression rate: 120 events/min (90 compressions interspersed with 30 ventilations).

Compression-ventilation ratio: 3:1 (pause compressions for ventilation).

Medications (epinephrine, volume): Indicated if heart rate remains <60/min despite adequate ventilation with 100% oxygen and chest compressions.

Estimation of Proper Endotracheal Tube Size and Depth of Insertion Based on Infant's Gestational Age and Weight

Weight (g)	Gestational Age (wk)	Laryngoscope Blade	Endotracheal Tube Size (mm)/ Catheter Size	Depth of Insertion From Upper Lip (cm)
Below 1000	<28	0	2.5/5F or 6F	6.5-7.0
1000-2000	28-34	0	3.0/6F or 8F	7.0-8.0
2000-3000	34-38	0-1	3.5/8F	8.0-9.0
>3000	>38	1	3.5-4.0/8F	>9.0

Medications Used During or Following Resuscitation of the Newborn

Medications	Dose/Route*	Concentration	Wt (kg)	Total IV Volume (mL)	Precautions
Epinephrine	IV (UVC preferred route) 0.01-0.03 mg/kg Higher IV doses not recommended Endotracheal up to 0.1 mg/kg	1:10 000	1 2 3 4	0.1-0.3 0.2-0.6 0.3-0.9 0.4-1.2	Give rapidly. Repeat every 3 to 5 minutes. Higher dose for endotracheal route may be needed (Class Indeterminate).
Volume expanders Isotonic crystalloid (normal saline) or blood	10 mL/kg IV		1 2 3 4	10 20 30 40	Indicated for shock. Give over 5 to 10 minutes. Reassess after each bolus.
Sodium bicarbonate (4.2% solution)	1 to 2 mEq/kg, IV	0.5 mEq/mL (4.2% solution)	1 2 3 4	2-4 4-8 6-12 8-16	Only for prolonged resuscitation. Use only if infant is effectively ventilated before administration. Give slow push, minimum 2 minutes.
Naloxone	0.1 mg/kg IV or IM preferred route Caution with SQ route Endotracheal route not recommended (Class Indeterminate)	0.4 mg/mL 1 mg/mL	1 2 3 4 1 2 3 4	0.25 0.50 0.75 1 0.1 0.2 0.3 0.4	Establish adequate ventilation first; not recommended for initial resuscitation. Give rapidly. Repeat every 2 to 3 minutes as needed (Class Indeterminate). Caution in opioid-addicted mothers.
Dextrose (10% solution)	0.2 g/kg, 2 mL/kg D_{10} IV	0.1 g/mL	1 2 3 4	2 4 6 8	Check bedside glucose. May require dilution from 25% or 50% dextrose using sterile water.

IV indicates intravenous; IM, intramuscular; SQ, subcutaneous; and UVC, umbilical vein catheter.
*Note: Endotracheal dose may not result in effective plasma concentration of drug, so vascular access should be established as soon as possible. Drugs given endotracheally require higher dosing and can be diluted to a total volume of 1 mL with normal saline before instillation; no clinical data regarding IO route of administration.

Pediatric Advanced Life Support

Primary cardiac arrest in children is much less common than in adults; **cardiac arrest in children typically results from progressive deterioration in cardiovascular or respiratory function.** The outcome of pediatric cardiac arrest remains poor, and emphasis must be placed on detection and appropriate treatment of respiratory failure, shock, and respiratory arrest and the prevention of progression to cardiac arrest.

Conditions Requiring Rapid Assessment and Potential Cardiopulmonary Support

- Respirations irregular or rate >60 breaths/min
- Heart rate ranges (particularly if associated with poor perfusion)
  - Child ≤2 years of age: <80/min or >180/min
  - Child >2 years of age: <60/min or >160/min
- Poor perfusion, with weak or absent distal pulses
- Increased work of breathing (retractions, nasal flaring, grunting)
- Cyanosis or a decrease in oxyhemoglobin saturation
- Altered level of consciousness (unusual irritability or lethargy or failure to respond to parents or painful procedures)
- Seizures
- Fever with petechiae
- Trauma
- Burns involving >10% of body surface area

Vital Signs in Children

Heart Rate (per minute)*

Age	Awake Rate	Mean	Sleeping Rate
Newborn to 3 months	85 to 205	140	80 to 160
3 months to 2 years	100 to 190	130	75 to 160
2 to 10 years	60 to 140	80	60 to 90
>10 years	60 to 100	75	50 to 90

Respiratory Rate (breaths/min)†

Age	Rate
Infant	30 to 60
Toddler	24 to 40
Preschooler	22 to 34
School-age child	18 to 30
Adolescent	12 to 16

Blood Pressure (BP)‡

- Typical systolic BP for 1 to 10 years of age (50th percentile): **90 + (age in years × 2) mm Hg**
- Lower limits of systolic BP for 1 to 10 years of age (5th percentile): **70 + (age in years × 2) mm Hg**
- Lower range of normal systolic BP for >10 years of age: **approximately 90 mm Hg**
- Typical mean arterial pressure (50th percentile): **55 + (age in years × 1.5) mm Hg**

---

*From Gillette PC, Garson A Jr, Porter CJ, McNamara DG. Dysrhythmias. In: Adams FH, Emmanouilides GC, Reimenschneider TA, eds. *Moss' Heart Disease in Infants, Children, and Adolescents.* 4th ed. Baltimore, Md: Williams & Wilkins; 1989:725-741.

†Reproduced from Hazinski MF. Children are different. In: Hazinski MF, ed. *Manual of Pediatric Critical Care.* St Louis, Mo: Mosby–Year Book; 1999.

‡Haque IU, Zaritsky AL. Analysis of the evidence for the lower limit of systolic and mean arterial pressure in children. *Pediatr Crit Care.* 2007; 8:138-144.

Assess-Categorize-Decide-Act (ACDA)

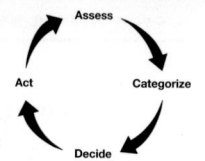

General Assessment

> If at any point during the general assessment you identify a life-threatening problem, immediately start lifesaving actions and get help!

Appearance	TICLS: Tone, Interactiveness, Consolability, Look/Gaze, Speech/Cry		
	All normal?	Any abnormal?	
Work of Breathing	Normal effort	Increased effort Decreased effort	Abnormal sounds
Circulation	Normal skin color, no external bleeding	Abnormal skin color	External bleeding
Not life threatening ➡ Go to primary assessment		Life threatening ➡ Act!	

Primary Assessment

> If at any point during the general assessment you identify a life-threatening problem, immediately start lifesaving actions and get help!

Airway	Clear			Maintainable		Not maintainable

Breathing	Respiratory Rate	Respiratory Effort	Air Movement	Airway and Breath Sounds		Pulse Oximetry
	Normal Fast Slow Apnea	Normal Nasal flaring Chest retractions Head bobbing Seesaw respirations	Normal Decreased	*Airway Sounds* Stridor Barking cough Grunting Gurgling	*Breath Sounds* Prolonged expiration Wheezing Crackles	Normal oxygen saturation Hypoxemia

Circulation	Heart Rate	Pulses		Capillary Refill Time	Skin Color, Temperature	Blood Pressure
	Normal Fast (tachycardia) Slow (bradycardia)	*Peripheral* Normal Weak Absent	*Central* Normal Weak Absent	Normal: 2 seconds or less Delayed: >2 seconds	Pale skin Mottling Cyanosis Warm skin Cool skin	Normal Abnormal

(continued)

Assess-Categorize-Decide-Act (ACDA) *(continued)*

Disability	AVPU Pediatric Response Scale				Pupil Size Reaction to Light		Blood Glucose	
	Alert	Responds to **V**oice	Responds to **P**ain	**U**nresponsive	Normal	Abnormal	Normal	Low

Exposure	Temperature			Skin	
	Normal	High	Low	Rash	Trauma

Categorize		
Problem	Type	Severity
Respiratory	Upper airway obstruction Lower airway obstruction Lung tissue disease Disordered control of breathing	Respiratory distress Respiratory failure

Circulatory	Hypovolemic shock Distributive shock Cardiogenic shock Obstructive shock	Compensated shock Hypotensive shock
Respiratory + Circulatory	Respiratory type(s) + Circulatory type(s)	Cardiopulmonary failure

Decide

Decide what to do

Act

Begin appropriate actions

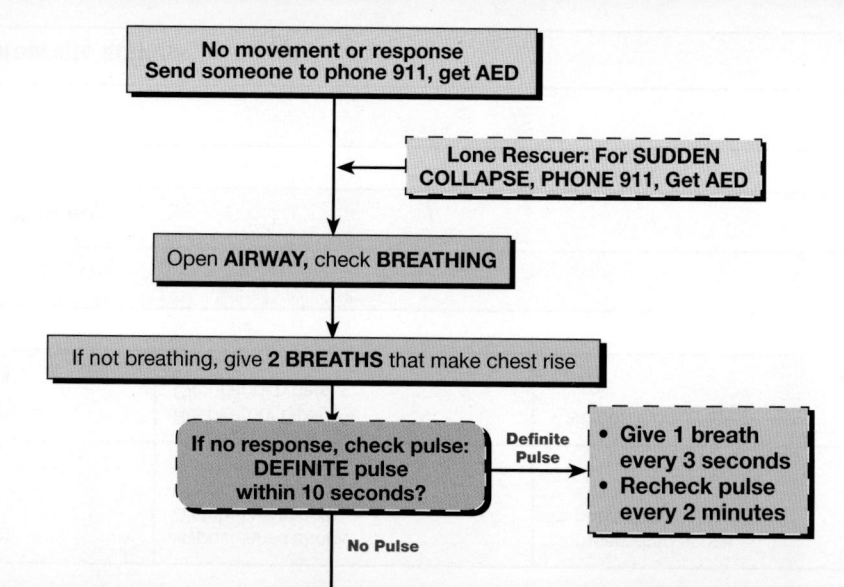

No movement or response
Send someone to phone 911, get AED

Lone Rescuer: For SUDDEN COLLAPSE, PHONE 911, Get AED

Open **AIRWAY,** check **BREATHING**

If not breathing, give **2 BREATHS** that make chest rise

If no response, check pulse: **DEFINITE** pulse within 10 seconds?

Definite Pulse
- Give 1 breath every 3 seconds
- Recheck pulse every 2 minutes

No Pulse

One Rescuer: Give cycles of **30 COMPRESSIONS** and **2 BREATHS**
Push hard and fast (100/min) and release completely
Minimize interruptions in compressions

Two Rescuers: Give cycles of **15 COMPRESSIONS** and **2 BREATHS**

⬇

If not already done, PHONE 911, for child get AED/defibrillator
Infant (<1 year): Continue CPR until ALS responders take over or
victim starts to move
Child (>1 year): Continue CPR; use AED/defibrillator after 2 minutes of CPR
(Use AED as soon as it is available for sudden, witnessed collapse)

⬇

Child >1 year:
Check rhythm
Shockable rhythm?

Shockable ← | → Not Shockable

Give 1 shock
Resume CPR immediately
for 2 minutes

Resume CPR immediately
for 2 minutes
Check rhythm every
2 minutes; continue until
ALS providers take over or
victim starts to move

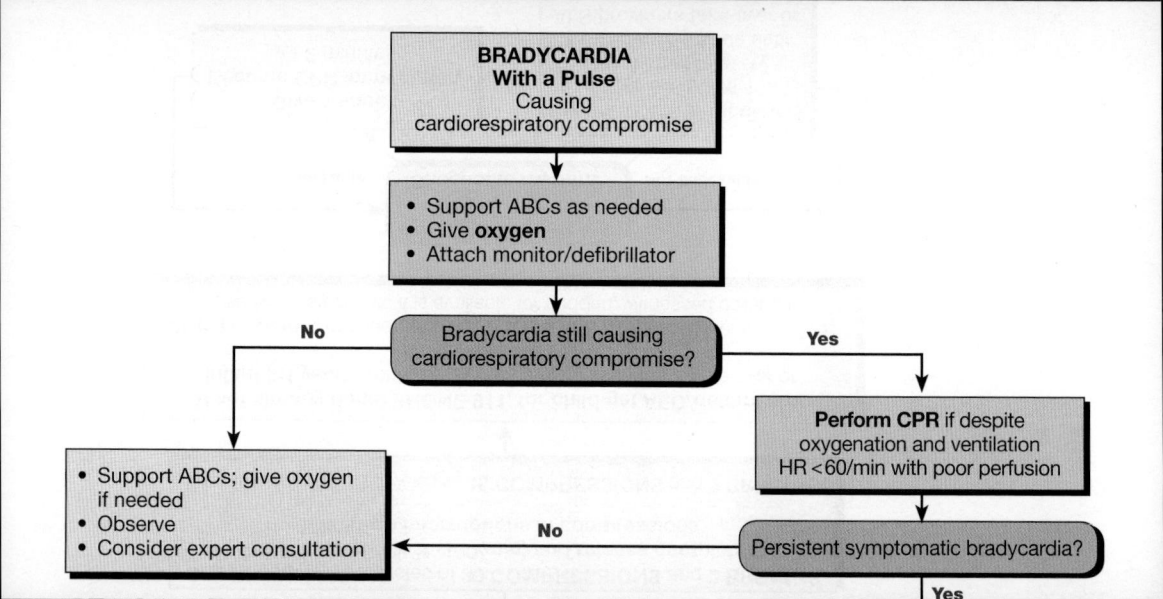

**BRADYCARDIA
With a Pulse**
Causing
cardiorespiratory compromise

- Support ABCs as needed
- Give **oxygen**
- Attach monitor/defibrillator

Bradycardia still causing cardiorespiratory compromise?

No

Yes

- Support ABCs; give oxygen if needed
- Observe
- Consider expert consultation

Perform CPR if despite oxygenation and ventilation HR <60/min with poor perfusion

No

Persistent symptomatic bradycardia?

Yes

Reminders

- **During CPR, push hard and fast (100/min)**

**Ensure full chest recoil
Minimize interruptions in
chest compressions**
- Support ABCs
- Secure airway if needed; confirm placement

- Search for and treat possible contributing factors:
  - **H**ypovolemia
  - **H**ypoxia or ventilation problems
  - **H**ydrogen ion (acidosis)
  - **H**ypo-/hyperkalemia
  - **H**ypoglycemia
  - **H**ypothermia
  - **T**oxins
  - **T**amponade, cardiac
  - **T**ension pneumothorax
  - **T**hrombosis (coronary or pulmonary)
  - **T**rauma (hypovolemia, increased ICP)

- **Give epinephrine**
  - IV/IO: 0.01 mg/kg (1:10 000: 0.1 mL/kg)
  - Endotracheal tube: 0.1 mg/kg (1:1000: 0.1 mL/kg)

  Repeat every 3 to 5 minutes

- **If increased vagal tone or primary AV block:** Give **atropine,** first dose: 0.02 mg/kg, may repeat. (Minimum dose: 0.1 mg; maximum total dose for child: 1 mg.)

- Consider cardiac pacing

If pulseless arrest develops, go to Pulseless Arrest Algorithm

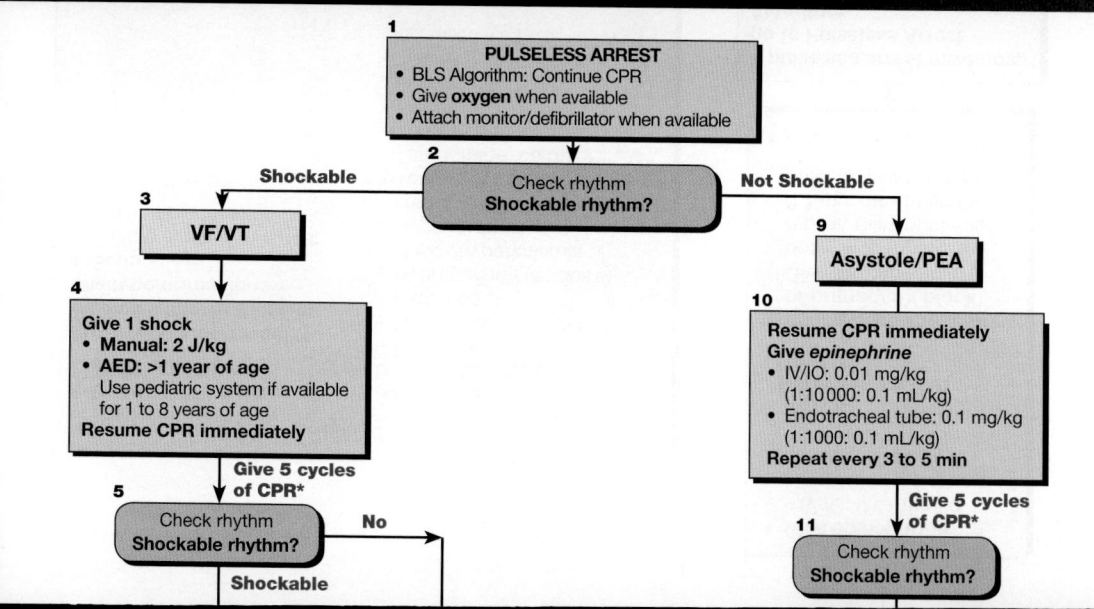

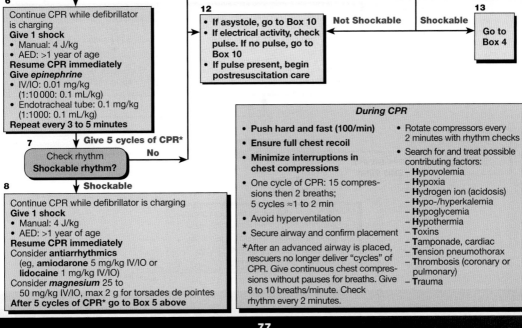

6

Continue CPR while defibrillator is charging
Give 1 shock
- Manual: 4 J/kg
- AED: >1 year of age
Resume CPR immediately
Give *epinephrine*
- IV/IO: 0.01 mg/kg
  (1:10 000: 0.1 mL/kg)
- Endotracheal tube: 0.1 mg/kg
  (1:1000: 0.1 mL/kg)
Repeat every 3 to 5 minutes

Give 5 cycles of CPR*

7

Check rhythm
Shockable rhythm?

No

Shockable

8

Continue CPR while defibrillator is charging
Give 1 shock
- Manual: 4 J/kg
- AED: >1 year of age
Resume CPR immediately
Consider **antiarrhythmics**
  (eg, **amiodarone** 5 mg/kg IV/IO or
  lidocaine 1 mg/kg IV/IO)
Consider *magnesium* 25 to
  50 mg/kg IV/IO, max 2 g for torsades de pointes
After 5 cycles of CPR* go to Box 5 above

12
- If asystole, go to Box 10
- If electrical activity, check pulse. If no pulse, go to Box 10
- If pulse present, begin postresuscitation care

Not Shockable   **Shockable**

13

Go to Box 4

During CPR

- **Push hard and fast (100/min)**
- **Ensure full chest recoil**
- **Minimize interruptions in chest compressions**
- One cycle of CPR: 15 compressions then 2 breaths; 5 cycles ≈1 to 2 min
- Avoid hyperventilation
- Secure airway and confirm placement

- Rotate compressors every 2 minutes with rhythm checks
- Search for and treat possible contributing factors:
  – **H**ypovolemia
  – **H**ypoxia
  – **H**ydrogen ion (acidosis)
  – **H**ypo-/hyperkalemia
  – **H**ypoglycemia
  – **H**ypothermia
  – **T**oxins
  – **T**amponade, cardiac
  – **T**ension pneumothorax
  – **T**hrombosis (coronary or pulmonary)
  – **T**rauma

*After an advanced airway is placed, rescuers no longer deliver "cycles" of CPR. Give continuous chest compressions without pauses for breaths. Give 8 to 10 breaths/minute. Check rhythm every 2 minutes.

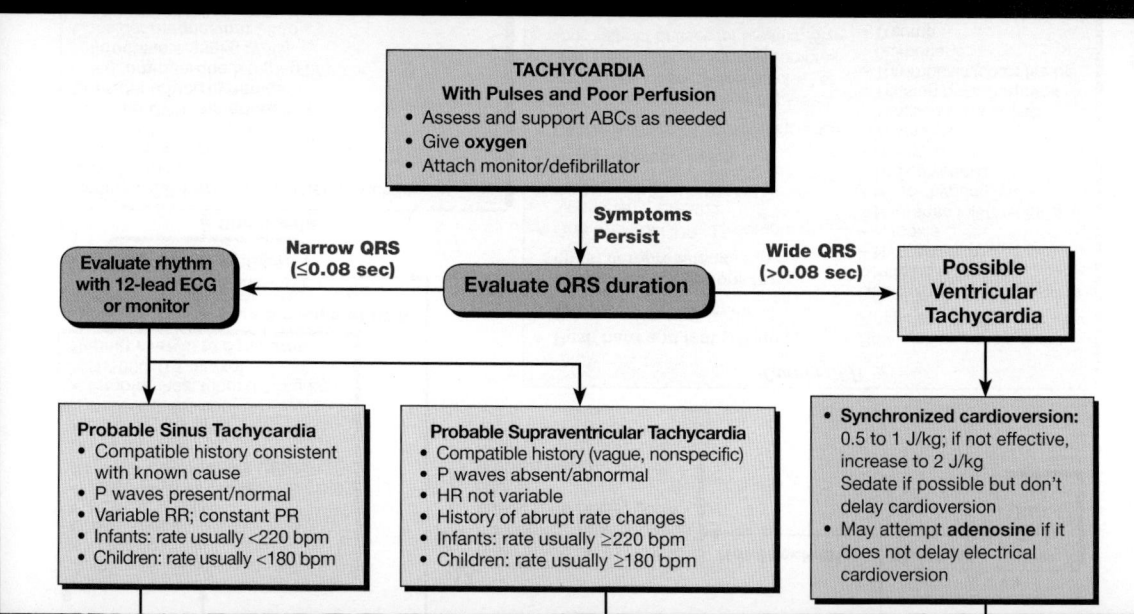

**TACHYCARDIA
With Pulses and Poor Perfusion**
- Assess and support ABCs as needed
- Give **oxygen**
- Attach monitor/defibrillator

Symptoms Persist

Evaluate QRS duration

Narrow QRS (≤0.08 sec)

Evaluate rhythm with 12-lead ECG or monitor

Wide QRS (>0.08 sec)

Possible Ventricular Tachycardia

Probable Sinus Tachycardia
- Compatible history consistent with known cause
- P waves present/normal
- Variable RR; constant PR
- Infants: rate usually <220 bpm
- Children: rate usually <180 bpm

Probable Supraventricular Tachycardia
- Compatible history (vague, nonspecific)
- P waves absent/abnormal
- HR not variable
- History of abrupt rate changes
- Infants: rate usually ≥220 bpm
- Children: rate usually ≥180 bpm

- Synchronized cardioversion: 0.5 to 1 J/kg; if not effective, increase to 2 J/kg
  Sedate if possible but don't delay cardioversion
- May attempt **adenosine** if it does not delay electrical cardioversion

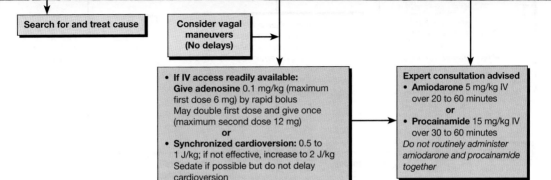

Search for and treat cause

Consider vagal maneuvers (No delays)

- If IV access readily available:
  Give adenosine 0.1 mg/kg (maximum first dose 6 mg) by rapid bolus
  May double first dose and give once (maximum second dose 12 mg)
  or
- **Synchronized cardioversion:** 0.5 to 1 J/kg; if not effective, increase to 2 J/kg
  Sedate if possible but do not delay cardioversion

Expert consultation advised
- **Amiodarone** 5 mg/kg IV over 20 to 60 minutes
  or
- **Procainamide** 15 mg/kg IV over 30 to 60 minutes
  Do not routinely administer amiodarone and procainamide together

During Evaluation	*Treat possible contributing factors:*	
• Secure, verify airway and vascular access when possible	– **H**ypovolemia	– **T**oxins
• Consider expert consultation	– **H**ypoxia	– **T**amponade, cardiac
	– **H**ydrogen ion (acidosis)	– **T**ension pneumothorax
• Prepare for cardioversion	– **H**ypo-/hyperkalemia	– **T**hrombosis (coronary or pulmonary)
	– **H**ypoglycemia	
	– **H**ypothermia	– **T**rauma (hypovolemia)

Pediatric Tachycardia With Adequate Perfusion Algorithm

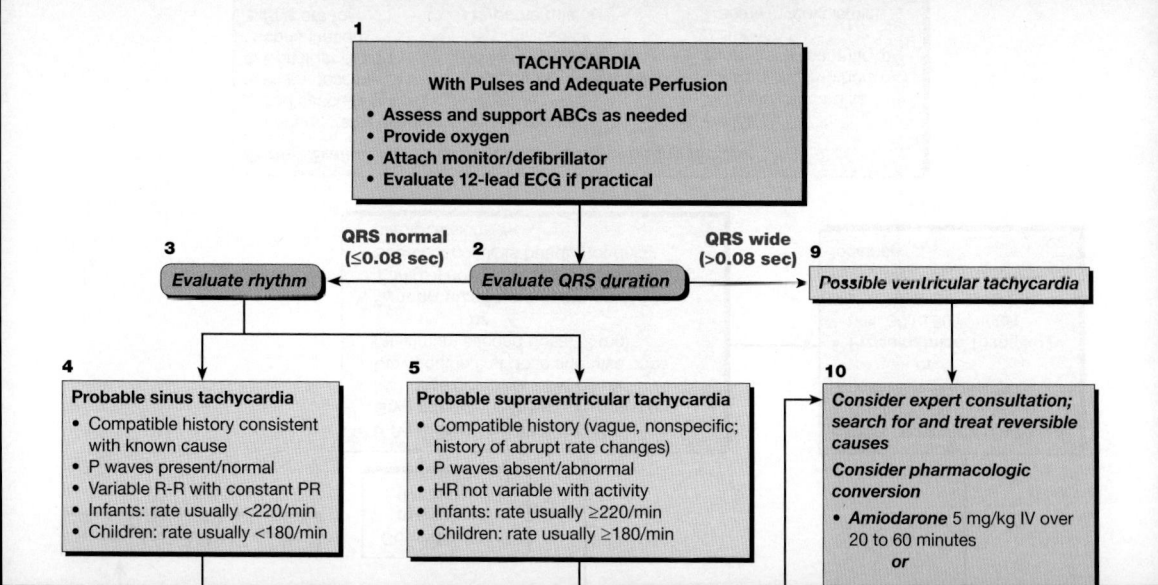

1

TACHYCARDIA
With Pulses and Adequate Perfusion

- Assess and support ABCs as needed
- Provide oxygen
- Attach monitor/defibrillator
- Evaluate 12-lead ECG if practical

2 *Evaluate QRS duration*

QRS normal (≤0.08 sec) →
3 *Evaluate rhythm*

QRS wide (>0.08 sec) →
9 *Possible ventricular tachycardia*

4

Probable sinus tachycardia
- Compatible history consistent with known cause
- P waves present/normal
- Variable R-R with constant PR
- Infants: rate usually <220/min
- Children: rate usually <180/min

5

Probable supraventricular tachycardia
- Compatible history (vague, nonspecific; history of abrupt rate changes)
- P waves absent/abnormal
- HR not variable with activity
- Infants: rate usually ≥220/min
- Children: rate usually ≥180/min

10

Consider expert consultation; search for and treat reversible causes

Consider pharmacologic conversion

- *Amiodarone* 5 mg/kg IV over 20 to 60 minutes
  or

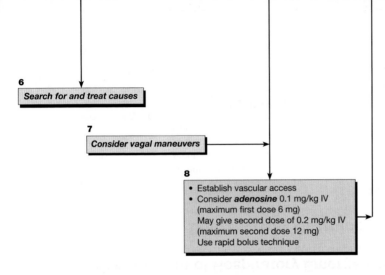

6

Search for and treat causes

7

Consider vagal maneuvers

8

- Establish vascular access
- Consider **adenosine** 0.1 mg/kg IV (maximum first dose 6 mg)
  May give second dose of 0.2 mg/kg IV (maximum second dose 12 mg)
  Use rapid bolus technique

- **Procainamide** 15 mg/kg IV over 30 to 60 minutes

Do not routinely administer amiodarone and procainamide together

- May attempt **adenosine** if not already administered

Consider electrical conversion

- Consult pediatric cardiologist
- Attempt **cardioversion** with 0.5 to 1 J/kg (may increase to 2 J/kg if initial dose ineffective)
- Sedate prior to cardioversion
- Obtain 12-lead ECG

Management of Respiratory Emergencies Flowchart

Management of Respiratory Emergencies Flowchart		
• Airway positioning • Oxygen • Pulse oximetry • ECG monitor (as indicated) • BLS as indicated		

Upper Airway Obstruction — Specific Management for Selected Conditions		
Croup	**Anaphylaxis**	**Aspiration Foreign Body**
• Nebulized epinephrine • Corticosteroids	• IM epinephrine (or auto-injector) • Albuterol • Antihistamines • Corticosteroids	• Allow position of comfort • Specialty consultation

Lower Airway Obstruction — Specific Management for Selected Conditions	
Bronchiolitis	**Asthma**
• Nasal suctioning • Bronchodilator trial	• Albuterol ± ipratropium • Magnesium sulfate • Corticosteroids • Terbutaline • SQ epinephrine

Lung Tissue (Parenchymal) Disease
Specific Management for Selected Conditions

Pneumonia/Pneumonitis _Infectious Chemical Aspiration_	**Pulmonary Edema** _Cardiogenic or Noncardiogenic (ARDS)_
• Albuterol • Antibiotics (as indicated)	• Consider noninvasive or invasive ventilatory support with PEEP • Consider vasoactive support • Consider diuretic

Disordered Control of Breathing
Specific Management for Selected Conditions

Increased ICP	_Poisoning/Overdose_	_Neuromuscular Disease_
• Avoid hypoxemia • Avoid hypercarbia • Avoid hyperthermia	• Antidote (if available) • Contact poison control	• Consider noninvasive or invasive ventilatory suport

Comparison of Steps in PALS and ACLS

Rapid Sequence Intubation Steps for PALS	Rapid Sequence Intubation Steps for ACLS
1. Brief medical history and focused physical assessment	
2. Preparation • Equipment • Personnel • Medications	1. Pre-event preparation
3. Monitoring	
4. Preoxygenation	2. Preoxygenation
5. Premedication	3. Pretreatment/Premedication
6. Sedation	4. Paralyze after sedation
7. Cricoid pressure and assisted ventilation (if needed)	5. Protection/Positioning
8. Neuromuscular blockade (pharmacologic paralysis)	
9. Endotracheal intubation	6. Placement of endotracheal tube
10. Postintubation monitoring and observation	7. Postintubation management
11. Continued sedation and paralysis	

Succinylcholine: Adverse Effects and Relative Contraindications

Adverse Effects	Relative Contraindications
Muscle pain	Increased intracranial pressure
Rhabdomyolysis	Open globe injury
Myoglobinuria	Glaucoma
Hyperkalemia	Neuromuscular disorders
Hypertension	History (patient or family) of malignant hyperthermia
Increased intracranial pressure	History of plasma cholinesterase deficiency
Increased intraocular pressure	Crush injuries
Increased intragastric pressure	Trauma or burns >48 hours after injury
Malignant hyperthermia	Hyperkalemia
Bradycardia/asystole	Renal failure

Pharmacologic Agents Used in Rapid Sequence Intubation for Children

Drug	Dose*	Route	Duration	Side Effects	Comments
Cardiovascular Adjuncts					
Atropine	IV: 0.01-0.02 mg/kg (minimum: 0.1 mg; maximum: 1 mg) IM: 0.02 mg/kg	IV, IM	>30 min	Paradoxical bradycardia can occur with doses <0.1 mg Tachycardia	Inhibits bradycardic response to hypoxia May cause pupil dilation but no evidence that it prevents pupil constriction to light
Glycopyrrolate Robinul®	0.005-0.01 mg/kg (maximum: 0.2 mg)	IV	>30 min	Tachycardia Dry mouth	Inhibits bradycardic response to hypoxia
Narcotic Agents					
Fentanyl citrate	2-4 µg/kg	IV, IM	IV 30-60 min IM 1-2 hours	Respiratory depression Hypotension Chest wall rigidity rarely with high-dose rapid infusions	Less histamine release and hypotension than with other opioids May lower BP and cause compensatory rise in ICP Movement disorders can occur with prolonged use

Sedative Hypnotic Agents					
Midazolam (Versed®)	0.1-0.2 mg/kg (maximum: 4 mg)	IV, IM	30-60 min	Respiratory depression Hypotension	Potentiates respiratory depressive effects of narcotics and barbiturates No analgesic properties
Diazepam (Valium®)	0.1-0.2 mg/kg (maximum: 4 mg)	IV	30-90 min		
Thiopental (Pentothal®)	2-5 mg/kg	IV	5-10 min	Negative inotropic effects Hypotension	Ultrashort-acting barbiturate Decreases cerebral metabolic rate and ICP Potentiates respiratory depressive effects of narcotics and benzodiazepines No analgesic properties
Etomidate	0.2-0.4 mg/kg **Caution:** limit to one dose; consider hydrocortisone stress doses for patients in shock	IV	10-15 min	Myoclonic activity Cortisol suppression	Ultrashort-acting No analgesic properties Decreases cerebral metabolic rate and ICP Minimal cardiovascular and respiratory depression Contraindicated in patients dependent on endogenous cortisol response

IM indicates intramuscular; CNS, central nervous system; ICP, intracranial pressure; and BP, blood pressure. *Doses provided are guidelines only. Actual dosing may vary, depending on patient's clinical status.

(continued on next page)

Pharmacologic Agents Used in Rapid Sequence Intubation for Children (continued)

Drug	Dose*	Route	Duration	Side Effects	Comments
Anesthetic Agents (when used in higher doses)					
Lidocaine	1-2 mg/kg	IV	≈30 min	Myocardial and CNS depression with high doses Seizures can occur with repeated doses	May decrease ICP during RSI Hypotension occurs infrequently
Ketamine	IV: 1-2 mg/kg IM: 3-5 mg/kg	IV, IM	30-60 min	Hypertension Increased secretions and laryngospasm Hallucinations Emergence reactions	Dissociative anesthetic agent Limited respiratory depression Bronchodilator Can cause myocardial depression in catecholamine-depleted patients (eg, those with chronic congestive heart failure or severe or prolonged shock)
Propofol (Diprovan®)	2 mg/kg (up to 3 mg/kg in young children)	IV	3-5 min	Hypotension, especially in patients with inadequate intravascular volume Pain on injection	Highly lipid soluble—very short duration of action Less airway reactivity than barbiturates

Neuromuscular Blocking Agents					
Succinylcholine	IV: 1-1.5 mg/kg for children IV: 2 mg/kg for infants IM: double the IV dose	IV, IM	3-5 min	May cause rhabdomyolysis Rise in intracranial, intraocular, intragastric pressure Life-threatening hyperkalemia Hypertension	Depolarizing muscle relaxant Rapid onset, short duration of action Avoid in renal failure, burns, crush injuries, hyperkalemia or family history of malignant hyperthermia Consider defasciculation with a nondepolarizing agent in children ≥5 years of age Do *not* use to maintain paralysis
Vecuronium (Norcuron®)	0.1-0.2 mg/kg	IV, IM	30-90 min	Minimal cardiovascular side effects	Nondepolarizing agent 2- to 3-min onset of action
Rocuronium (Zemuron®)	0.6-1.2 mg/kg	IV	30-60 min	Minimal cardiovascular side effects	Nondepolarizing agent Rapid onset of action

IM indicates intramuscular; CNS, central nervous system; ICP, intracranial pressure; and BP, blood pressure.

*Doses provided are guidelines only. Actual dosing may vary, depending on patient's clinical status.

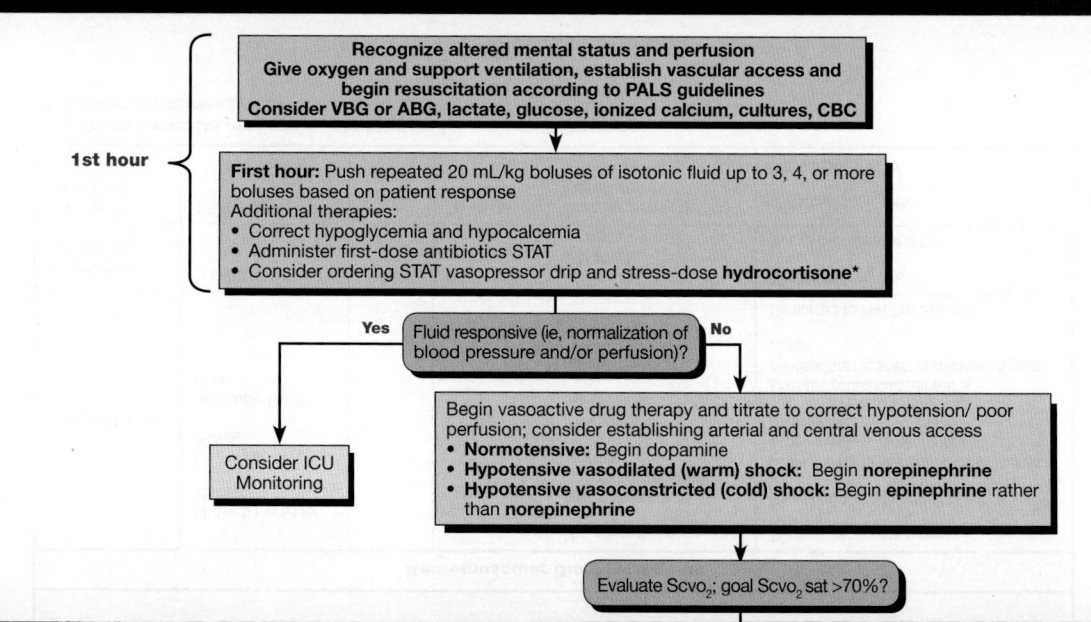

Recognize altered mental status and perfusion
Give oxygen and support ventilation, establish vascular access and begin resuscitation according to PALS guidelines
Consider VBG or ABG, lactate, glucose, ionized calcium, cultures, CBC

1st hour

First hour: Push repeated 20 mL/kg boluses of isotonic fluid up to 3, 4, or more boluses based on patient response
Additional therapies:
- Correct hypoglycemia and hypocalcemia
- Administer first-dose antibiotics STAT
- Consider ordering STAT vasopressor drip and stress-dose **hydrocortisone***

Yes ← Fluid responsive (ie, normalization of blood pressure and/or perfusion)? → **No**

Consider ICU Monitoring

Begin vasoactive drug therapy and titrate to correct hypotension/ poor perfusion; consider establishing arterial and central venous access
- **Normotensive:** Begin dopamine
- **Hypotensive vasodilated (warm) shock:** Begin norepinephrine
- **Hypotensive vasoconstricted (cold) shock:** Begin epinephrine rather than norepinephrine

Evaluate $Scvo_2$; goal $Scvo_2$ sat >70%?

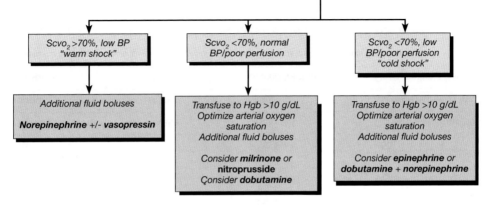

$Scvo_2$ >70%, low BP "warm shock"

$Scvo_2$ <70%, normal BP/poor perfusion

$Scvo_2$ <70%, low BP/poor perfusion "cold shock"

Additional fluid boluses

Norepinephrine +/- **vasopressin**

Transfuse to Hgb >10 g/dL
Optimize arterial oxygen saturation
Additional fluid boluses

Consider **milrinone** or **nitroprusside**
Consider **dobutamine**

Transfuse to Hgb >10 g/dL
Optimize arterial oxygen saturation
Additional fluid boluses

Consider **epinephrine** or **dobutamine** + **norepinephrine**

*Note: Fluid refractory and dopamine- or norepinephrine-dependent shock defines patient at risk for adrenal insufficiency.

Draw baseline cortisol; consider ACTH stimulation test if unsure of need for steroids

If adrenal insufficiency is suspected give **hydrocortisone** ~2 mg/kg bolus IV; maximum 100 mg

Modified from Parker MM, Hazelzet JA, Carcillo JA. Pediatric considerations. *Crit Care Med.* 2004;32:S591-S594.

Pediatric Trauma Score

Patient Characteristics	Category Value		
	+2	+1	−1
Weight (kg)	>20	10 to 20	<10
Airway	Normal	Maintained	Unable to maintain
Systolic blood pressure (mm Hg)	>90	50 to 90	<50
Central nervous system	Awake	Obtunded	Coma/decerebrate posture
Open wound	None	Minor	Major/penetrating trauma
Skeletal trauma	None	Closed fractures	Open, multiple fractures

Add the value for each patient characteristic. Highest possible total score is +12, and lowest possible total score is −6.

From Tepas JJ III, Mollitt DL, Talbert JL, Bryant M. The pediatric trauma score as a predictor of injury severity in the injured child. *J Pediatr Surg*. 1987:22:14-18.

Categorization of Hemorrhage and Shock in Pediatric Trauma Patients Based on Systemic Signs of Decreased Organ and Tissue Perfusion

System	Mild Hemorrhage, Compensated Shock, Simple Hypovolemia (<30% blood volume loss)	Moderate Hemorrhage, Decompensated Shock, Marked Hypovolemia (30%-45% blood volume loss)	Severe Hemorrhage, Cardiopulmonary Failure, Profound Hypovolemia (>45% blood volume loss)
Cardiovascular	Mild tachycardia Weak peripheral pulses, strong central pulses Low-normal blood pressure (SBP >70 mm Hg + [2 × age in y]) Mild acidosis	Moderate tachycardia Thready peripheral pulses, weak central pulses Frank hypotension (SBP <70 mm Hg + [2 × age in y]) Moderate acidosis	Severe tachycardia Absent peripheral pulses, thready central pulses Profound hypotension (SBP <50 mm Hg) Severe acidosis
Respiratory	Mild tachypnea	Moderate tachypnea	Severe tachypnea
Neurologic	Irritable, confused	Agitated, lethargic	Obtunded, comatose
Integumentary	Cool extremities, mottling Poor capillary refill (>2 seconds)	Cool extremities, pallor Delayed capillary refill (>3 seconds)	Cold extremities, cyanosis Prolonged capillary refill (>5 seconds)
Excretory	Mild oliguria, increased specific gravity	Marked oliguria, increased blood urea nitrogen	Anuria

SBP indicates systolic blood pressure.

Used/Reproduced with permission from American College of Surgeons' Committee on Trauma, from *Advanced Trauma Life Support ® for Doctors (ATLS ®) Student Manual, 2004 (7th) Edition,* American College of Surgeons. Chicago: First Impressions.

**Approach to Fluid Resuscitation
in Child With Multiple Injuries**

Signs of inadequate systemic perfusion are present*

↓

Rapid infusion (<20 minutes) 20 mL/kg of NS or LR

↓

Continued signs of inadequate systemic perfusion?

Yes

↓

Second rapid infusion 20 mL/kg of NS or LR

↓

Continued signs of inadequate systemic perfusion?

Approach to the Child With Multiple Injuries

Note: Effective trauma resuscitation requires a team effort. The assessments and interventions below may be performed simultaneously.

1. Before arrival, notify *trauma surgeon with pediatric expertise*.

2. Open airway with jaw thrust, maintaining manual cervical spine stabilization.

3. Clear the oropharynx with a rigid suction device; assess breathing.

4. Administer 100% oxygen by nonrebreathing mask if child is responsive and breathing spontaneously.

5. Ventilate with bag-mask and 100% oxygen if child has inadequate respiratory effort or respiratory distress or is unresponsive. Hyperventilate only if there are signs of impending brain herniation.

6. Provide advanced airway management with appropriate manual cervical spine stabilization if the child has signs of respiratory failure or is unresponsive. Trained healthcare providers may attempt endotracheal intubation; confirm endotracheal tube placement with clinical assessment and a device (eg, exhaled CO_2 detector, esophageal detector device).

Yes ↓

- **Third rapid infusion 20 mL/kg of NS or LR**

  or

- **Packed RBCs (10 mL/kg), mixed with NS, bolus**

  Repeat every 20 to 30 minutes, as needed

*In child with severe trauma and life-threatening blood loss:
- Blood for STAT type and crossmatch
- Use 0-negative blood in females and 0-positive or 0-negative blood in males.

If the victim is unconscious during bag-mask ventilation, consider use of an oropharyngeal airway and cricoid pressure.

7. While maintaining airway patency and spine stabilization, assess signs of circulation.

8. Initiate chest compressions and control external bleeding with direct pressure if indicated.

9. Treat tension pneumothorax via needle decompression.

10. Establish vascular access; obtain blood samples for blood type and crossmatch studies.

11. Rapidly infuse 20 mL/kg isotonic crystalloid for inadequate perfusion.

12. Immobilize the neck with a semirigid collar, head immobilizer, and tape. In prehospital settings, immobilize thighs, pelvis, shoulders, and head to long spine board.

13. Consider gastric decompression (an orogastric tube is preferred if head trauma present).

14. Infuse a second isotonic crystalloid bolus if signs of shock are present. Consider blood products for major hemorrhage.

15. Consider need for surgical exploration if hypotension is present on arrival or if hemodynamic instability persists despite crystalloid and blood administration.

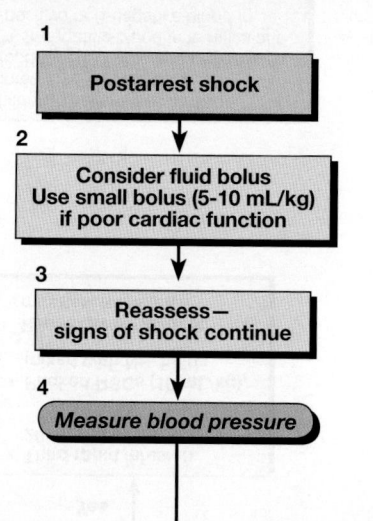

1
Postarrest shock

2
Consider fluid bolus
Use small bolus (5-10 mL/kg)
if poor cardiac function

3
Reassess—
signs of shock continue

4
Measure blood pressure

Estimation of Maintenance Fluid Requirements

- Infants <10 kg: Infusion of D_5 normal saline after initial stabilization at a rate of 4 mL/kg per hour. For example, the maintenance rate for an 8-kg baby is as follows:

  4 mL/kg per hour × 8 kg = 32 mL/h

- Children 10 to 20 kg: Infusion of 0.9% sodium chloride (normal saline) after initial stabilization at a rate of 40 mL/h plus 2 mL/kg per hour for each kilogram between 10 and 20 kg. For example, the maintenance rate for a 15-kg child is as follows:

  40 mL/h +

  (2 mL/kg per hour × 5 kg) =

  50 mL/h

Hypotensive shock? | Normotensive shock?

5

Consider further fluid boluses

and

- **Epinephrine** (0.1 to 1 µg/kg per minute)

and/or

- **Dopamine** begin at higher doses (10 to 20 µg/kg per minute)

and/or

- **Norepinephrine** (0.1 to 2 µg/kg per minute)

6

Consider further fluid boluses
and

- **Dobutamine** (2 to 20 µg/kg per minute)

and/or

- **Dopamine** (2 to 20 µg/kg per minute)

and/or

- Low-dose **epinephrine** (0.05 to 0.3 µg/kg per minute)

and/or

- ***Inamrinone***: Load with 0.75 to 1 mg/kg over 5 minutes, may repeat up to 3 mg/kg. Infusion: 5 to 10 µg/kg per minute. *Note: Inamrinone replaced by Milrinone in Canada.

or

- **Milrinone**: Load with 50 to 75 µg/kg over 10 to 60 minutes. Infusion: 0.5 to 0.75 µg/kg per minute.

- Children >20 kg: Infusion of 0.9% sodium chloride (normal saline) after initial stabilization at a rate of 60 mL/h plus 1 mL/kg per hour for each kilogram above 20 kg. For example, the maintenance rate for a 30-kg child is as follows:

$$60 \text{ mL/h} +$$

$$(1 \text{ mL/kg per hour} \times 10 \text{ kg}) =$$

$$70 \text{ mL/h}$$

- Shortcut for patients weighing >20 kg:

$$\text{weight in kg} + 40 \text{ mL/h}$$

Adjust rate and composition of fluids to child's clinical condition (eg, pulse, blood pressure, systemic perfusion) and level of hydration.

Pediatric Resuscitation Supplies*
Based on Color-Coded Resuscitation Tape

PALS

Equipment	GREY* 3-5 kg	PINK Small Infant 6-7 kg	RED Infant 8-9 kg	PURPLE Toddler 10-11 kg	YELLOW Small Child 12-14 kg	WHITE Child 15-18 kg	BLUE Child 19-23 kg	ORANGE Large Child 24-29 kg	GREEN Adult 30-36 kg
Resuscitation bag		Infant/child	Infant/child	Child	Child	Child	Child	Child	Adult
O$_2$ mask (NRB)**		Pediatric	Pediatric	Pediatric	Pediatric	Pediatric	Pediatric	Pediatric	Pediatric/adult
Oral airway (mm)		50	50	60	60	60	70	80	80
Laryngoscope blade (size)		1 straight	1 straight	1 straight	2 straight	2 straight	2 straight or curved	2 straight or curved	3 straight or curved
ET tube (mm)†		3.5 uncuffed	3.5 uncuffed	4.0 uncuffed	4.5 uncuffed	5.0 uncuffed	5.5 uncuffed	6.0 cuffed	6.5 cuffed
ET tube insertion length (cm)	3 kg 9-9.5 4 kg 9.5-10 5 kg 10-10.5	10.5-11	10.5-11	11-12	13.5	14-15	16.5	17-18	18.5-19.5
Stylet (F)		6	6	6	6	6	14	14	14
Suction catheter (F)		8	8	10	10	10	10	10	10-12
BP cuff	Neonatal #5/Infant	Infant/child	Infant/child	Child	Child	Child	Child	Child	Small adult
IV catheter (Ga)		22-24	22-24	20-24	18-22	18-22	18-20	18-20	16-20
IO (Ga)		18/15	18/15	15	15	15	15	15	15
NG tube (F)		5–8	5-8	8-10	10	10	12-14	14-18	16-18
Urinary catheter (F)	5	8	8	8-10	10	10-12	10-12	12	12
Chest tube (F)		10-12	10-12	16-20	20-24	20-24	24-32	28-32	32-38

*For Grey column, use Pink or Red equipment sizes if no size is listed. NRB is nonrebreather; ET, endotracheal.

†Per *2005 AHA Guidelines*, in the in-hospital setting cuffed or uncuffed tubes may be used (see below for sizing of cuffed tubes).

Adapted from *Broselow™ Pediatric Emergency Tape*, copyright 2007 Vital Signs, Inc. Distributed by Armstrong Medical Industries, Lincolnshire, Illinois.

Estimating Endotracheal Tube Size and Depth of Insertion

Tube Size

Several formulas such as the ones below allow estimation of proper endotracheal tube size (ID, internal diameter) for children 1 to 10 years of age, based on the child's age:

Uncuffed endotracheal tube size (mm ID) = (age in years/4) + 4

During preparation for intubation, providers also should have ready at the bedside uncuffed endotracheal tubes 0.5 mm smaller and larger than that estimated from the above formula.

The formula for estimation of a cuffed endotracheal tube size is as follows:

Cuffed endotracheal tube size (mm ID) = (age in years/4) + 3

Depth of Insertion

The formula for estimation of depth of insertion (measured at the lip) can be estimated from the child's age or the tube size.

Depth of insertion (cm) for children >2 years of age = (age in years/2) + 12

or the following:

Depth of insertion = tube internal diameter (mm) × 3

Confirm placement with both clinical assessment (eg, breath sounds, chest expansion) and device (eg, exhaled CO_2 detector or esophageal detector device). Watch for marker on endotracheal tube at vocal cords.

*Khine HH, Corddry DH, Kettrick RG, Martin TM, McCloskey JJ, Rose JB, Theroux MC, Zagnoev M. Comparison of cuffed and uncuffed endotracheal tubes in young children during general anesthesia. *Anesthesiology*. 1997;86:627–631; discussion 27A.

Administration Notes

Peripheral Intravenous (IV):	Resuscitation drugs administered via peripheral IV catheter should be followed by a bolus of at least 5 mL NS to move drug into central circulation.
Intraosseous (IO):	Drugs that can be administered by IV route may be administered by IO route. They should be followed by a bolus of at least 5 mL NS to move drug into central circulation.
Endotracheal:	Drugs that can be administered by endotracheal route are indicated in the tables below. **IV/IO administration is preferred** because it provides more reliable drug delivery and pharmacologic effect. For some drugs the optimum endotracheal doses have not been established. Doses given by ET route should generally be higher than standard IV doses. For infants and children, dilute the medication with NS to a volume of 3 to 5 mL, instill in the endotracheal tube and follow with flush of 3 to 5 mL. Provide 5 positive-pressure breaths after medication is instilled.
Continuous infusion:	Infusion rate (mL/h) = $\dfrac{\text{Weight (kg)} \times \text{dose (µg/kg per minute)} \times 60 \text{ min/h}}{\text{Concentration (µg/mL)}}$

Drug/Therapy	Indications/Precautions	Pediatric Dosage
Adenosine	**Indications** Drug of choice for treatment of symptomatic SVT. **Precautions** Very short half-life.	**IV/IO Administration** • 0.1 mg/kg *rapid* IV push • **Maximum first dose: 6 mg.** • **Maximum single dose: 12 mg.** • Follow immediately with 5 to 10 mL NS flush. • May give 0.2 mg/kg for second dose. **Maximum second dose: 12 mg.** • Continuous ECG monitoring. **Injection Technique** • Record rhythm strip during administration. • Draw up adenosine dose and flush (5 to 10 mL) in 2 separate syringes. • Attach both syringes to the IV injection port closer to patient. • Clamp IV tubing above injection port. • Push IV adenosine as *quickly* as possible (1 to 3 seconds). • While maintaining pressure on adenosine plunger, push NS flush *as rapidly as possible* after adenosine. • Unclamp IV tubing.

Drug/Therapy	Indications/Precautions	Pediatric Dosage
Albuterol Nebulized solution: 0.5% (5 mg/mL) Prediluted nebulized solution: 0.63 mg/3 mL NS, 1.25 mg/3 mL NS, 2.5 mg/3 mL NS (0.083%) MDI: 90 µg/puff	**Indications** Bronchodilator, β_2-adrenergic agent • Asthma • Anaphylaxis (bronchospasm) • Hyperkalemia	**For Asthma, Anaphylaxis (mild to moderate), Hyperkalemia** • **MDI (q 20 min)** —4 to 8 puffs (inhalation) PRN with spacer • **Nebulizer (q 20 min)** —Weight <20 kg: 2.5 mg/dose (inhalation) —Weight >20 kg: 5 mg/dose (inhalation) **For Asthma, Anaphylaxis (severe)** • **Continuous nebulizer** —0.5 mg/kg per hour continuous inhalation (maximum dose 20 mg/h) • **MDI** (recommended if intubated) —4 to 8 puffs (inhalation) via ETT q 20 minutes PRN or with spacer if not intubated

Alprostadil (PGE$_1$)
See Prostaglandin E$_1$ (PGE$_1$)

Amiodarone

Indications
Can be used for treatment of atrial and ventricular arrhythmias in children, particularly ectopic atrial tachycardia, junctional ectopic tachycardia, and ventricular tachycardia.

Precautions
- May produce hypotension. May prolong QT interval and increase propensity for polymorphic ventricular arrhythmias. Therefore, routine administration in combination with procainamide is not recommended without expert consultation.
- Use with caution if hepatic failure is present.
- Terminal elimination is extremely long (elimination half-life with chronic oral dosing is up to 40 days).

For Refractory VF, Pulseless VT
5 mg/kg IV/IO bolus; can repeat the 5 mg/kg IV/IO bolus up to total dose of 15 mg/kg (2.2 g in adolescents) IV per 24 hours.
Maximum single dose: 300 mg.

For Perfusing Supraventricular and Ventricular Arrhythmias
Loading dose: 5 mg/kg IV/IO over 20 to 60 minutes (maximum single dose: 300 mg). Can repeat to maximum of 15 mg/kg (2.2 g in adolescents) per day IV.

Drug/Therapy	Indications/Precautions	Pediatric Dosage

Atropine Sulfate
 	
Can be given by endotracheal tube
	Indications
	• Symptomatic bradycardia (usually secondary to vagal stimulation)
	• Toxins/overdose (eg, organophosphate, carbamate).
	• Rapid sequence intubation (RSI): (ie, age <1 year, age 1 to 5 years receiving succinylcholine, age >5 years receiving second dose of succinylcholine)
	
	Precautions
	• Contraindicated in angle closure glaucoma, tachyarrhythmias, thyrotoxicosis
	• Drug blocks bradycardic response to hypoxia. Monitor with pulse oximetry.
		Symptomatic Bradycardia
		• **IV/IO:** 0.02 mg/kg (min dose: 0.1 mg)
		  – Max single dose for child: 0.5 mg
		    for adolescent: 1 mg
		  – May repeat dose once.
		  – Max total dose for child: 1 mg
		    for adolescent: 2 mg
		  – Larger doses may be needed for organophosphate poisoning.
		• **ET:** 0.04 to 0.06 mg/kg
		
		Toxins/Overdose
		• <12 years: 0.02 to 0.05 mg/kg IV/IO initially, then repeated IV/IO q 20 to 30 minutes until muscarinic symptoms reverse
		• >12 years: 0.05 mg/kg IV/IO initially, then 1 to 2 mg IV/IO q 20 to 30 minutes until muscarinic symptoms reverse
		
		RSI
		IV/IO: 0.01 to 0.02 mg/kg (min dose: 0.1 mg, max dose: 1 mg)
		IM: 0.02 mg/kg

Calcium Chloride

10% = 100 mg/mL =
27.2 mg/mL elemental
calcium

Indications
- Treatment of documented or suspected conditions:
  - Hypocalcemia
  - Hyperkalemia
- Consider for treatment of
  - Hypermagnesemia
  - Calcium channel blocker overdose

Precautions
- Do not use routinely during resuscitation (may contribute to cellular injury).
- Not recommended for routine treatment of asystole or pulseless electrical activity.
- Rapid IV administration may cause hypotension, bradycardia, or asystole (particularly if patient is receiving digoxin).
- Do not mix with or infuse immediately before or after sodium bicarbonate without intervening flush.

IV/IO Administration
- 20 mg/kg (0.2 mL/kg) slow IV/IO push.
- May repeat if documented or suspected clinical indication persists (eg, toxicologic problem)
- Central venous administration preferred if available.

Drug/Therapy	Indications/Precautions	Pediatric Dosage

Calcium Gluconate
 	
10% = 100 mg/mL = 9 mg/mL elemental calcium
	Indications
	• Treatment of documented or suspected conditions:
	  — Hypocalcemia
	  — Hyperkalemia
	• Consider for treatment of:
	  — Hypermagnesemia
	  — Calcium channel blocker overdose
	
	Precautions
	• Do not use routinely during resuscitation (may contribute to cellular injury).
	• Not recommended for routine treatment of asystole or pulseless electrical activity.
	• Rapid IV administration may cause hypotension, bradycardia, or asystole (particularly if patient is receiving digoxin).
	• Do not mix with or infuse immediately before or after sodium bicarbonate without intervening flush.
		IV/IO Administration
		• 60 to 100 mg/kg (0.6 to 1 mL/kg) slow IV/IO push.
		• May repeat if documented or suspected clinical indication persists (eg, toxicologic problem).
		• Central venous administration preferred if available.

Cardioversion (Synchronized)

Indications
Treatment of choice for patients with evidence of cardiovascular compromise and tachyarrhythmias (SVT, VT, atrial fibrillation, or atrial flutter).

Precautions
- Synchronized (sync) mode must be activated. If severe hypotension or decompensated shock is present, intubation and ventilation with 100% oxygen and establishment of vascular access are desirable, but these therapies should not delay cardioversion. "Clear" before cardioversion.
- Consider sedation if patient is conscious and time and clinical condition allow.
- Consider metabolic or toxic cause of arrhythmias if they persist despite shocks.

- Make sure "sync" button is activated before shock.
- Initial energy level: 0.5 to 1 J/kg.*
- Second and subsequent energy levels: 2 J/kg.*
- If rhythm does not convert, reevaluate rhythm.

Note: In 2005 there was insufficient evidence to recommend a different dose for biphasic versus monophasic waveform shocks.

Drug/Therapy	Indications/Precautions	Pediatric Dosage
Corticosteroids	**Precautions** Use for more than a few days can cause hypertension, hyperglycemia, and increased risk of gastric bleeding.	
Dexamethasone	**Indications** • Croup (mild to severe) • Asthma (mild to moderate) • Vasogenic cerebral edema (eg, from brain tumor or abscess)	**Dexamethasone** **For Croup** • **Moderate to severe** —0.6 mg/kg PO/IM/IV × 1 dose (maximum dose 16 mg) • **Impending respiratory failure** —0.6 mg/kg IV (maximum dose 16 mg) **For Asthma** • **Mild to moderate** —0.6 mg/kg PO/IM/IV q 24 hours × 2 doses (maximum dose 16 mg) **For Vasogenic Cerebral Edema** • 1 to 2 mg/kg IV/IO *load*, then 1 to 1.5 mg/kg per day divided every 4 to 6 hours (maximum daily dose 16 mg)

Hydrocortisone	**Indications** Treatment of adrenal insufficiency (may be associated with septic shock).	**Hydrocortisone** **Adrenal Insufficiency** 2 mg/kg IV/IO bolus (maximum dose 100 mg).
Methylprednisolone	**Indications** • Ashtma (status asthmaticus) • Anaphylactic shock	**Methylprednisolone** **Status Asthmaticus, Anaphylactic Shock** • Load: 2 mg/kg IV/IO/IM (maximum 80 mg). *Note:* Must use acetate salt IM. • Maintenance: 0.5 mg/kg IV q 6 hours or 1 mg/kg q 12 hours up to 120 mg/day
Dobutamine	**Indications** Treatment of shock associated with high systemic vascular resistance (eg, congestive heart failure or cardiogenic shock). Ensure adequate intravascular volume. **Precautions** • May produce or exacerbate hypotension. • May produce tachyarrhythmias. • Do not mix with sodium bicarbonate. • Extravasation may cause tissue injury.	**Continuous IV/IO Infusion** • Titrate to desired effect. Typical infusion dose: 2 to 20 μg/kg per minute.

Drug/Therapy	Indications/Precautions	Pediatric Dosage
Dopamine	**Indications** Treatment of shock with adequate intravascular volume and stable rhythm. **Precautions** • High infusion rates (>20 µg/kg per minute) may cause splanchnic vasoconstriction, ischemia. • May produce tachyarrhythmias. • Do not mix with sodium bicarbonate. • Extravasation may cause tissue injury. • May affect thyroid function.	**Continuous IV/IO Infusion** • Titrate to desired effect. Typical infusion dose: 2 to 20 µg/kg per minute. ***Note:*** If infusion dose >20 µg/kg per minute is required, consider using alternative adrenergic agent (eg, epinephrine).

Epinephrine

Standard: 1:10 000 or
0.1 mg/mL

High: 1:1000 or
1 mg/mL

Can be given via
endotracheal tube

Indications
- Bolus IV therapy
  - Treatment of pulseless arrest.
  - Treatment of symptomatic bradycardia unresponsive to O_2 and ventilation.
- Continuous IV infusion
  - Shock (poor perfusion) or hypotension in patient with adequate intravascular volume and stable rhythm.
  - Clinically significant bradycardia.
  - β-Blocker or calcium channel blocker overdose.
  - Pulseless arrest when bolus therapy fails.

Precautions
- May produce tachyarrhythmias.
- High-dose infusions may produce vasoconstriction, may compromise perfusion; low doses may decrease renal and splanchnic blood flow.
- Do not mix with sodium bicarbonate.
- Correct acidosis, hypoxemia.
- Contraindicated in treatment of VT secondary to cocaine (may be considered if VF develops).

Pulseless Arrest
- **IV/IO dose:** 0.01 mg/kg (0.1 mL/kg of 1:10 000 standard concentration). Administer every 3 to 5 minutes during arrest (maximum dose of 1 mg).
- **All endotracheal doses:** 0.1 mg/kg (0.1 mL/kg of 1:1000 high concentration).
  - Administer every 3 to 5 minutes of arrest until IV/IO access achieved; then begin with first IV dose.

Symptomatic Bradycardia
- **All IV/IO doses:** 0.01 mg/kg (0.1 mL/kg of 1:10 000 standard concentration).
- **All endotracheal doses:** 0.1 mg/kg (0.1 mL/kg of 1:1000 high concentration).

Continuous IV/IO Infusion
Once tubing is primed, titrate to response. Typical initial infusion: 0.1 to 1 μg/kg per minute. Higher doses may be effective.

Drug/Therapy	Indications/Precautions	Pediatric Dosage
Etomidate	**Indications** • Ultrashort-acting nonbarbiturate, non-benzodiazepine sedative-hypnotic agent with no analgesic properties. • Produces rapid sedation with no untoward cardiovascular or respiratory depression. • Sedative of choice for multiple trauma or hypotensive patients. • Decreases ICP, cerebral blood flow, and cerebral basal metabolic rate; recommended for sedation of head-injured patients. **Precautions** • May suppress cortisol production after a single dose. Consider administration of stress dose hydrocortisone (2 mg/kg; maximum dose 100 mg). • May also cause myoclonic activity (coughing, hiccups) and may exacerbate focal seizure disorders. • Relative contraindications include known adrenal insufficiency or history of focal seizure disorder.	**For Rapid Sedation** • IV/IO dose of 0.2 to 0.4 mg/kg infused over 30 to 60 seconds will produce rapid sedation that lasts 10 to 15 minutes. • Maximum dose: 20 mg.

Glucose

Indications
Treatment of hypoglycemia (documented or strongly suspected).

Precautions
- Use bedside glucose test to confirm hypoglycemia; hyperglycemia may worsen neurologic outcome of cardiopulmonary arrest or trauma; do not administer routinely during resuscitation.
- Maximum concentration for newborn administration: 12.5% (0.125 g/mL).

IV/IO Infusion
- 0.5 to 1 g/kg (maximum recommended IV/IO concentration: 25%; can prepare by mixing 50% dextrose 1:1 with sterile water).
  - **50%** dextrose (0.5 g/mL); give 1 to 2 mL/kg.
  - **25%** dextrose (0.25 g/mL); give 2 to 4 mL/kg.
  - **10%** dextrose (0.1 g/mL); give 5 to 10 mL/kg.
  - **5%** dextrose (0.05 g/mL); give 10 to 20 mL/kg if volume tolerated.

---

*Inamrinone

(Amrinone)

*Note: Inamrinone has been replaced by Milrinone in Canada.

Indications
Myocardial dysfunction and increased systemic or pulmonary vascular resistance, including
- Congestive heart failure in postoperative cardiovascular surgical patients.
- Shock with high systemic vascular resistance.

Precautions
- May produce hypotension, particularly in volume-depleted patients.
- Long elimination half-life.
- May increase platelet destruction.
- Drug may accumulate in renal failure and in patients with low cardiac output.

Loading Dose
0.75 to 1 mg/kg IV/IO over 5 minutes; may repeat twice (maximum: 3 mg/kg).

Continuous Infusion
5 to 10 µg/kg per minute IV/IO.

Caution: Do not dilute in dextrose solution but can be co-infused with dextrose solutions.

Drug/Therapy	Indications/Precautions	Pediatric Dosage
Ipratropium Bromide	**Indications** Anticholinergic and bronchodilator used for treatment of asthma **Precautions** • May cause pupil dilation if it enters eyes.	**Inhalation Dose** • 250 to 500 µg (by nebulizer, MDI) q 20 minutes × 3 doses.
Lidocaine Can be given via endotracheal tube	**Indications** • Bolus therapy: — VF/pulseless VT. — Wide-complex tachycardia (with pulses). • Rapid sequence intubation (RSI): May decrease ICP response during laryngoscopy. **Precautions/Contraindications** • High plasma concentration may cause myocardial and circulatory depression, possible CNS symptoms (eg, seizures). • Reduce infusion dose if severe CHF or low cardiac output is compromising hepatic and renal blood flow. • Contraindicated for bradycardia with wide-complex ventricular escape beats.	**VF/Pulseless VT, Wide-Complex Tachycardia (With Pulses)** **IV/IO:** • Initial: 1 mg/kg IV/IO loading dose. • Maintenance: 20 to 50 µg/kg per minute IV/IO infusion (repeat bolus dose if infusion initiated >15 minutes after initial bolus therapy). **ET:** 2 to 3 mg/kg. **Rapid Sequence Intubation (RSI)** 1 to 2 mg/kg IV/IO

Magnesium Sulfate

50% = 500 mg/mL

Indications
- Torsades de pointes or suspected hypomagnesemia.
- Status asthmaticus not responsive to β-adrenergic drugs.

Precautions/Contraindications
- Contraindicated in renal failure.
- Possible hypotension and bradycardia with rapid bolus.

Pulseless VT With Torsades
25 to 50 mg/kg IV/IO bolus (maximum dose: 2 g).

Torsades (With Pulses), Hypomagnesemia
25 to 50 mg/kg IV/IO (maximum dose: 2 g) over 10 to 20 minutes.

Status Asthmaticus
25 to 50 mg/kg IV/IO over 15 to 30 minutes; (maximum dose: 2 g).

Drug/Therapy	Indications/Precautions	Pediatric Dosage
Naloxone Can be given by IV/IO/IM/SQ Endotracheal route possible; other routes preferred	**Indications** To reverse effects of narcotic toxicity: respiratory depression, hypotension, and hypoperfusion. **Precautions** • Half-life of naloxone often shorter than half-life of narcotic; repeated dosing is often required. • Administration to infants of addicted mothers may precipitate seizures or other withdrawal symptoms. • Assist ventilation before naloxone administration to avoid sympathetic stimulation. • May reverse effects of analgesics; consider administration of non-opioid analgesics for treatment of pain.	**Bolus IV/IO Dose** For *total* reversal of narcotic effects give 0.1 mg/kg q 2 minutes PRN (maximum dose 2 mg). ***Note:*** If total reversal is not required (eg, respiratory depression), smaller doses (1 to 5 μg/kg) may be used. Titrate to effect. **Continuous IV/IO Infusion** 0.002 to 0.16 mg/kg per hour IV/IO infusion.

Nitroprusside
(Sodium Nitroprusside)

Mix in D_5W

Vasodilator that reduces tone in all vascular beds.

Indications
- Shock or low cardiac output states (cardiogenic shock) characterized by high vascular resistance.
- Severe hypertension.

Precautions
- May cause hypotension, particularly with hypovolemia.
- Metabolized by endothelial cells to cyanide, then metabolized in liver to thiocyanate and excreted by kidneys. Thiocyanate and cyanide toxicity may result if administered at high rates or with decreased hepatic or renal function. Monitor thiocyanate levels in patients receiving prolonged infusion, particularly if rate >2 µg/kg per minute.
- Signs of thiocyanate toxicity include seizures, nausea, vomiting, metabolic acidosis, and abdominal cramps.

IV/IO Infusion
- Children ≤40 kg: 1 to 8 µg/kg per minute. *Note:* Some references recommend beginning infusions at 0.3 µg/kg per minute.
- Children >40 kg: 0.1 to 5 µg/kg per minute.
- Light-sensitive; cover drug reservoir with opaque material or use specialized administration set.
- Typically change the solution every 24 hours.

Pediatric Advanced Life Support Drugs and Electrical Therapy

PALS

Drug/Therapy	Indications/Precautions	Pediatric Dosage
Norepinephrine	Sympathetic neurotransmitter with potent inotropic effects. Activates myocardial β-adrenergic receptors and vascular α-adrenergic receptors. **Indications** Treatment of shock and hypotension characterized by low systemic vascular resistance and unresponsive to fluid resuscitation. **Precautions** • May produce hypertension, organ ischemia, and arrhythmias. Extravasation may cause tissue necrosis (treat with phentolamine). • Do not administer in same IV tubing with alkaline solutions.	Begin at rates of 0.1 to 2 µg/kg per minute; adjust infusion rate to achieve desired change in blood pressure and systemic perfusion.
Oxygen	**Indications** • Should be administered during stabilization of all seriously ill or injured patients with respiratory insufficiency, shock, or trauma even if oxyhemoglobin saturation is normal. • May monitor pulse oximetry to evaluate oxygenation and titrate therapy once child has adequate perfusion.	• Administer in highest possible concentration during initial evaluation and stabilization. • A nonrebreathing mask with reservoir delivers 95% oxygen with flow rate of 10 to 15 L/min.

Procainamide

Indications
SVT, atrial flutter, VT (with pulses).

Precautions
- Seek expert consultation when using this agent.
- Routine use in combination with amiodarone (or other drugs that prolong QT interval) is not recommended without expert consultation.
- Risk of hypotension and negative inotropic effects increases with rapid administration; not appropriate agent for VF/pulseless VT.
- Reduce dose for patients with poor renal or cardiac function.

Loading Dose
15 mg/kg IV/IO over 30 to 60 minutes.

Prostaglandin E₁ (PGE₁)

Indications
To maintain patency of ductus arteriosus in newborns with cyanotic congenital heart disease and ductal-dependent pulmonary or systemic blood flow.

Precautions
- May produce vasodilation, hypotension, apnea, hyperpyrexia, agitation, seizures.
- May produce hypoglycemia, hypocalcemia.

IV/IO Administration

Initial
0.05 to 0.1 µg/kg per minute IV/IO infusion.

Maintenance
0.01 to 0.05 µg/kg per minute IV/IO infusion.

Drug/Therapy	Indications/Precautions	Pediatric Dosage
Sodium Bicarbonate 8.4%: 1 mEq/mL in 10- or 50-mL syringe 4.2%: 0.5 mEq/mL in 10-mL syringe	**Indications** • Treatment of severe metabolic acidosis (documented or following prolonged arrest) unresponsive to ventilation and oxygenation. • Treatment of the following: — Hyperkalemia. — Sodium channel blocker toxicity, such as tricyclic antidepressants (after support of adequate airway and ventilation). **Precautions** • Infuse slowly. • Buffering action will produce carbon dioxide, so ventilation must be adequate. • Do not mix with any resuscitation drugs. Flush IV tubing with NS before and after drug administration. • Infiltration will cause tissue irritation.	**IV/IO Administration** **Metabolic Acidosis (Severe), Hyperkalemia** IV/IO: 1 mEq/kg *slow* bolus. 4.2% concentration recommended for use in infants <1 month of age. **Sodium Channel Blocker Overdose (eg, Tricyclic Antidepressant)** 1 to 2 mEq/kg IV/IO bolus until serum pH is >7.45 (7.50 to 7.55 for severe poisoning) followed by IV/IO infusion of 150 mEq $NaHCO_3$/L solution to maintain alkalosis.

Nitroprusside
(Sodium Nitroprusside)

Mix in D_5W

Vasodilator that reduces tone in all vascular beds.

Indications
- Shock or low cardiac output states (cardiogenic shock) characterized by high vascular resistance.
- Severe hypertension.

Precautions
- May cause hypotension, particularly with hypovolemia.
- Metabolized by endothelial cells to cyanide, then metabolized in liver to thiocyanate and excreted by kidneys. Thiocyanate and cyanide toxicity may result if administered at high rates or with decreased hepatic or renal function. Monitor thiocyanate levels in patients receiving prolonged infusion, particularly if rate >2 µg/kg per minute.
- Signs of thiocyanate toxicity include seizures, nausea, vomiting, metabolic acidosis, and abdominal cramps.

IV/IO Infusion
- Children ≤40 kg: 1 to 8 µg/kg per minute. *Note:* Some references recommend beginning infusions at 0.3 µg/kg per minute.
- Children >40 kg: 0.1 to 5 µg/kg per minute.
- Light-sensitive; cover drug reservoir with opaque material or use specialized administration set.
- Typically change the solution every 24 hours.

Drug/Therapy	Indications/Precautions	Pediatric Dosage
Norepinephrine	Sympathetic neurotransmitter with potent inotropic effects. Activates myocardial β-adrenergic receptors and vascular α-adrenergic receptors. **Indications** Treatment of shock and hypotension characterized by low systemic vascular resistance and unresponsive to fluid resuscitation. **Precautions** • May produce hypertension, organ ischemia, and arrhythmias. Extravasation may cause tissue necrosis (treat with phentolamine). • Do not administer in same IV tubing with alkaline solutions.	Begin at rates of 0.1 to 2 µg/kg per minute; adjust infusion rate to achieve desired change in blood pressure and systemic perfusion.
Oxygen	**Indications** • Should be administered during stabilization of all seriously ill or injured patients with respiratory insufficiency, shock, or trauma even if oxyhemoglobin saturation is normal. • May monitor pulse oximetry to evaluate oxygenation and titrate therapy once child has adequate perfusion.	• Administer in highest possible concentration during initial evaluation and stabilization. • A nonrebreathing mask with reservoir delivers 95% oxygen with flow rate of 10 to 15 L/min.

Procainamide

Indications
SVT, atrial flutter, VT (with pulses).

Precautions
- Seek expert consultation when using this agent.
- Routine use in combination with amiodarone (or other drugs that prolong QT interval) is not recommended without expert consultation.
- Risk of hypotension and negative inotropic effects increases with rapid administration; not appropriate agent for VF/pulseless VT.
- Reduce dose for patients with poor renal or cardiac function.

Loading Dose
15 mg/kg IV/IO over 30 to 60 minutes.

Prostaglandin E$_1$ (PGE$_1$)

Indications
To maintain patency of ductus arteriosus in newborns with cyanotic congenital heart disease and ductal-dependent pulmonary or systemic blood flow.

Precautions
- May produce vasodilation, hypotension, apnea, hyperpyrexia, agitation, seizures.
- May produce hypoglycemia, hypocalcemia.

IV/IO Administration

Initial
0.05 to 0.1 µg/kg per minute IV/IO infusion.

Maintenance
0.01 to 0.05 µg/kg per minute IV/IO infusion.

Drug/Therapy	Indications/Precautions	Pediatric Dosage

Sodium Bicarbonate

8.4%: 1 mEq/mL in 10- or 50-mL syringe

4.2%: 0.5 mEq/mL in 10-mL syringe

Indications
- Treatment of severe metabolic acidosis (documented or following prolonged arrest) unresponsive to ventilation and oxygenation.
- Treatment of the following:
  — Hyperkalemia.
  — Sodium channel blocker toxicity, such as tricyclic antidepressants (after support of adequate airway and ventilation).

Precautions
- Infuse slowly.
- Buffering action will produce carbon dioxide, so ventilation must be adequate.
- Do not mix with any resuscitation drugs. Flush IV tubing with NS before and after drug administration.
- Infiltration will cause tissue irritation.

IV/IO Administration

Metabolic Acidosis (Severe), Hyperkalemia
IV/IO: 1 mEq/kg *slow bolus.*

4.2% concentration recommended for use in infants <1 month of age.

Sodium Channel Blocker Overdose (eg, Tricyclic Antidepressant)
1 to 2 mEq/kg IV/IO bolus until serum pH is >7.45 (7.50 to 7.55 for severe poisoning) followed by IV/IO infusion of 150 mEq $NaHCO_3$/L solution to maintain alkalosis.